MANAGING HEART DISEASE THROUGH DIET

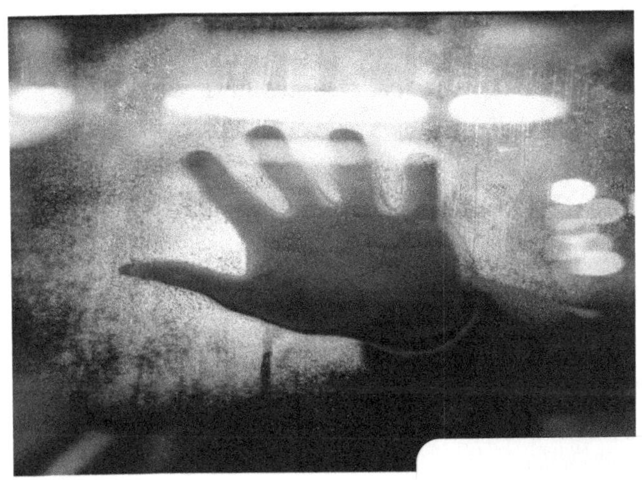

"Nutritional Strategies for Heart Disease Management"

Emma Lynch

TABLE OF CONTENTS

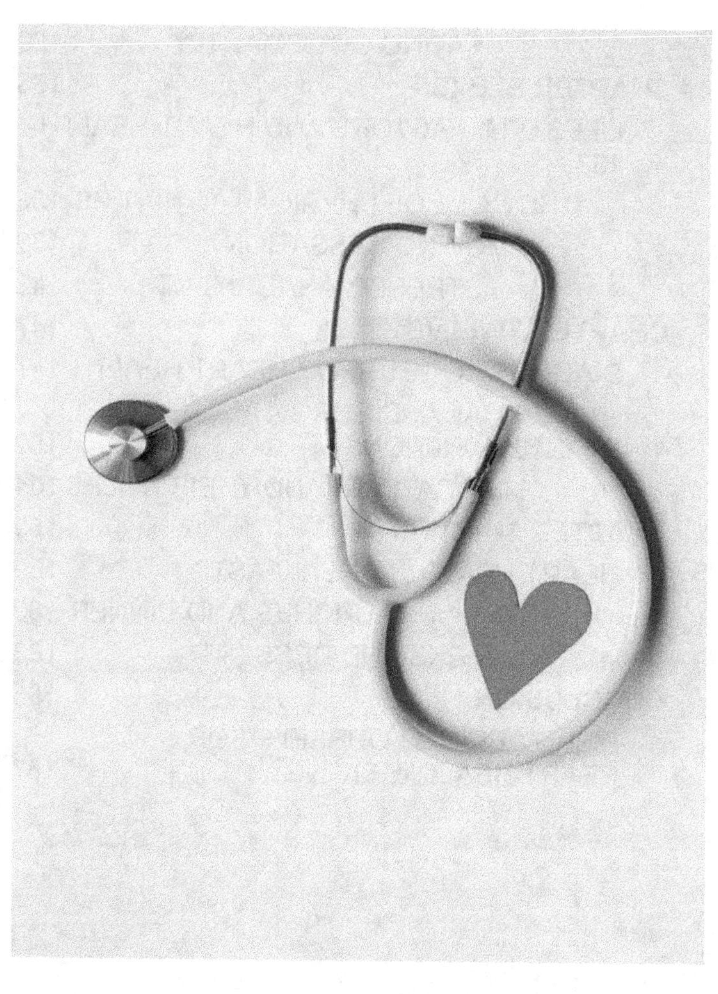

INTRODUCTION

In an era where the pace of modern life often leads to dietary choices that are less than optimal, heart disease has emerged as a major public health challenge. Heart disease, encompassing conditions like coronary artery disease, congestive heart failure, and hypertension, remains a leading cause of mortality globally. The good news is that many of the risk factors associated with heart disease, including unhealthy dietary habits, are within our control.

Diet plays a pivotal role in the development and management of heart disease. What we choose to eat, how we prepare our meals, and the nutritional content of our diets can significantly impact our cardiovascular health. With the right knowledge and mindful dietary choices, it is possible to not only reduce the risk of heart disease but also manage its effects for those already diagnosed.

This comprehensive guide is designed to delve deep into the intricate relationship between diet and heart health. We will explore the science behind heart disease, dissect the components of a heart-healthy diet, and offer practical strategies for incorporating these dietary changes into your daily life. Our aim is to empower you with the information and tools needed to make informed dietary decisions that will contribute to a healthier heart and a better quality of life.

So, join us on this journey to discover the profound impact of nutrition on cardiovascular wellness and equip yourself with the knowledge and skills necessary to manage heart disease through diet effectively.

CHAPTER ONE

UNDERSTANDING HEART DISEASE

Heart disease, which is another name for cardiovascular illness, is a collection of disorders affecting the heart and blood arteries. It is one of the main causes of death in the globe. To understand heart disease, it's important to break it down into several key components:

1. Types of Heart Disease:
  - **Coronary Artery Disease (CAD):** This is the most common type of heart disease and occurs when the blood vessels supplying the heart muscle become narrow or blocked. Heart attacks or angina (chest pain) may result from it.
  - **Heart Failure:** Heart failure doesn't mean the heart has stopped beating, but rather that it can't pump blood effectively, causing fatigue, shortness of breath, and fluid retention.
  - **Arrhythmias:** These are irregular heart rhythms, which can lead to palpitations, dizziness, or fainting.
  - **Valvular Heart Disease:** This involves issues with the heart valves, such as narrowing (stenosis) or leaking (regurgitation), which can affect blood flow.

2. Risk Factors:
   - **Modifiable Risk Factors:** These include lifestyle factors like an unhealthy diet, lack of physical activity, smoking, and excessive alcohol consumption. These can be changed through lifestyle modifications.
   - **Non-Modifiable Risk Factors:** These include age, family history, and genetics. While these can't be changed, awareness of them is important for early detection and management.

3. Prevention:
   - Heart disease can often be prevented or mitigated through a heart-healthy lifestyle. This includes eating a balanced diet low in saturated and trans fats, maintaining a healthy weight, regular physical activity, managing stress, not smoking, and limiting alcohol intake.

4. Diagnosis and Treatment:
   - Early diagnosis is critical for effective treatment. It typically involves medical history, physical exams, and tests like electrocardiograms (ECGs), echocardiograms, and blood tests.
   - Treatment options may include lifestyle changes, medications, medical procedures, or surgery, depending on the specific condition and its severity.

5. Ongoing Management:
   - For those with heart disease, ongoing management is crucial. This may involve

medication, lifestyle adjustments, and regular medical check-ups to monitor progress and make necessary changes.

Understanding heart disease is the first step in taking control of your heart health. By adopting a heart-healthy lifestyle and working closely with healthcare professionals, individuals can reduce their risk of heart disease and effectively manage its impact on their lives.

IMPORTANCE OF DIET IN MANAGING HEART HEALTH

Diet plays a central role in managing heart health. It's not just about counting calories or losing weight; it's about making informed food choices to protect your heart and overall well-being. Here are some key reasons why diet is essential in managing heart health:

1. **Control of Risk Factors:** A heart-healthy diet can help manage and control risk factors associated with heart disease, such as high blood pressure, high cholesterol levels, and diabetes. By reducing these risk factors, you can significantly lower your chances of developing heart disease.

2. **Cholesterol Management:** A diet low in saturated and trans fats can help lower "bad" LDL cholesterol levels, which contribute to the buildup of

plaque in the arteries. This, in turn, reduces the risk of atherosclerosis (narrowing of the arteries) and related heart conditions.

3. **Blood Pressure Regulation:** A diet rich in fruits, vegetables, whole grains, and low in sodium can help regulate blood pressure. High blood pressure is a major risk factor for heart disease, and a heart-healthy diet can contribute to its control.

4. **Weight Management:** Maintaining a healthy weight through diet is crucial for heart health. Excess body weight can strain the heart, increase blood pressure, and lead to conditions like obesity and type 2 diabetes.

5. **Inflammation Reduction:** Certain foods, like those rich in antioxidants and omega-3 fatty acids, can help reduce inflammation in the body. Chronic inflammation is associated with the development of heart disease.

6. **Prevention of Plaque Buildup:** A diet high in fiber, particularly soluble fiber, can help prevent the buildup of plaque in the arteries by reducing the absorption of cholesterol in the bloodstream.

7. **Balanced Blood Sugar:** A heart-healthy diet can help manage blood sugar levels, which is crucial for individuals with diabetes or those at risk

of developing it. Heart disease is a substantial risk factor in diabetes.

8. **Improvement in Overall Health:** A diet focused on whole, nutrient-dense foods provides essential vitamins, minerals, and antioxidants that not only protect your heart but also contribute to your overall health and well-being.

9. **Lifestyle Integration:** A heart-healthy diet is a long-term lifestyle choice, and it often goes hand in hand with other heart-protective habits such as regular physical activity, not smoking, and managing stress.

In summary, a heart-healthy diet is a cornerstone of managing heart health. It can help control risk factors, reduce the chances of heart disease development, and improve overall health. Consulting with a healthcare professional or registered dietitian can be a valuable step in creating a personalized dietary plan that aligns with your specific needs and goals.

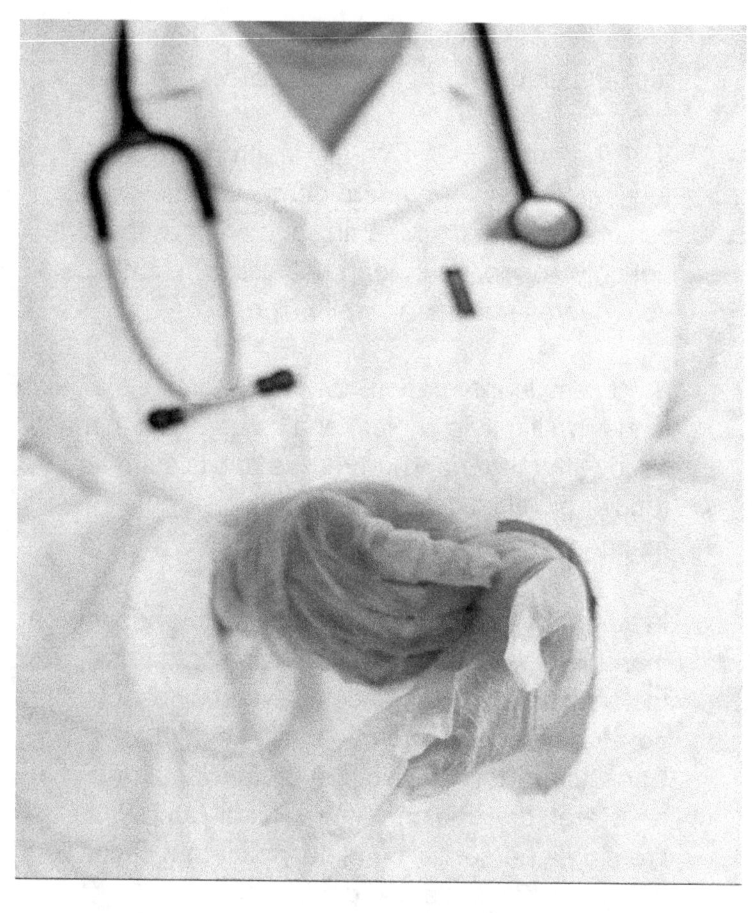

CHAPTER TWO

TYPES OF HEART DISEASE

There are several types of heart disease, each with its own characteristics and impact on the heart's function. Here are some examples of the most common types:

1. **Coronary Artery Disease (CAD):** CAD is the most prevalent type of heart disease. It occurs when the blood vessels (coronary arteries) that supply the heart muscle become narrow or blocked due to the buildup of plaque. This can lead to chest pain (angina) or, if the blood supply is severely restricted or cut off, a heart attack.

2. **Heart Failure:** Heart failure doesn't mean the heart has stopped beating, but rather that it can't pump blood effectively. This can result in fatigue, shortness of breath, and fluid retention. Heart failure can be caused by various conditions, including CAD, high blood pressure, and heart valve problems.

3. **Arrhythmias:** Arrhythmias are irregular heart rhythms. They may show up as an irregular, too fast, or too slow heartbeat. While some arrhythmias are harmless, others can be life-threatening and may lead to conditions like palpitations, dizziness, or fainting.

4. **Valvular Heart Disease:** This type of heart disease involves issues with the heart valves. Heart valves can become narrowed (stenosis) or leaky (regurgitation). Valvular heart disease can affect blood flow through the heart and may require surgical intervention to repair or replace the affected valve.

5. **Cardiomyopathy:** Cardiomyopathy is a condition where the heart muscle becomes weak and unable to pump blood effectively. It can be inherited or caused by various factors, including high blood pressure, viral infections, and excessive alcohol consumption.

6. **Congenital Heart Disease:** This refers to heart defects that are present at birth. These defects can affect the structure and function of the heart, leading to a wide range of heart conditions. Some congenital heart diseases are mild, while others are complex and may require surgery or other treatments.

7. **Peripheral Artery Disease (PAD):** PAD is a condition where there is a reduced blood flow to the limbs, usually the legs, due to atherosclerosis. While not a heart disease in the traditional sense, it is closely related because it involves the narrowing of blood vessels.

8. **Rheumatic Heart Disease:** This condition can result from untreated strep throat or scarlet fever. It can lead to heart valve damage and heart failure.

9. **Infective Endocarditis:** This is an infection of the heart's inner lining or the heart valves. It can be caused by bacteria or other microorganisms and may damage the heart valves.

Each type of heart disease requires different diagnostic and treatment approaches, but they all share the common importance of managing risk factors through a heart-healthy lifestyle and, in many cases, dietary changes.

CORONARY ARTERY DISEASE (CAD)

Coronary Artery Disease, often referred to as CAD, is the most common type of heart disease and a leading cause of heart-related health issues. It is primarily characterized by the narrowing or blockage of the coronary arteries, the blood vessels that supply the heart muscle with oxygen and nutrients.

Causes and Risk Factors:

The primary cause of CAD is the buildup of plaque within the coronary arteries. Plaque is made up of cholesterol, fatty substances, calcium, and other materials. Over time, this plaque can harden and narrow the arteries, a process known as atherosclerosis. The following risk factors are involved in the development of CAD:

- **High Cholesterol:** Elevated levels of low-density lipoprotein (LDL) cholesterol can increase the buildup of plaque in the arteries.
- **High Blood Pressure:** Hypertension can damage the artery walls, making them more susceptible to plaque buildup.
- **Smoking:** Smoking is a significant risk factor as it damages the arteries and reduces the amount of oxygen that can reach the heart.
- **Diabetes:** High blood sugar levels can contribute to atherosclerosis.
- **Obesity:** Excess body weight can lead to conditions like diabetes and hypertension.
- **Physical Inactivity:** A sedentary lifestyle can increase the risk of CAD.
- **Unhealthy Diet:** Diets high in saturated and trans fats, as well as excessive salt and sugar, can contribute to the development of CAD.

Symptoms:

The symptoms of CAD can vary and may include:

- Angina: Chest pain or discomfort, often triggered by physical activity or emotional stress.
- Shortness of breath: Especially during physical exertion.

- Fatigue: Feeling unusually tired, which may occur with or without chest discomfort.

In some cases, CAD can progress to a heart attack (myocardial infarction), which can cause severe chest pain, shortness of breath, and other life-threatening symptoms.

Diagnosis:

CAD is typically diagnosed through a combination of medical history, physical examination, and various tests, including electrocardiograms (ECGs or EKGs), stress tests, and coronary angiography.

Treatment:

Treatment for CAD may involve a combination of lifestyle changes, medications, and medical procedures. Lifestyle changes often include adopting a heart-healthy diet, increasing physical activity, quitting smoking, and managing stress. Drugs can aid in the management of risk factors like elevated blood pressure and cholesterol. In more severe cases, medical procedures like angioplasty and stent placement or coronary artery bypass surgery may be necessary to restore blood flow to the heart.

Managing CAD is a long-term commitment, and individuals with this condition often need ongoing medical care to reduce their risk of complications and improve their heart health.

HEART FAILURE

A chronic medical illness known as heart failure occurs when the heart is unable to adequately pump blood to meet the body's needs. It's often a progressive condition and can be caused by various factors, including coronary artery disease, high blood pressure, heart valve disease, and other heart conditions.

Types of Heart Failure:

1. **Systolic Heart Failure:** In this type, the heart's left ventricle becomes weakened and cannot contract effectively, reducing its ability to pump blood.

2. **Diastolic Heart Failure:** This type occurs when the left ventricle becomes stiff and cannot fill with blood properly during the resting phase between heartbeats.

Causes and Risk Factors:

Heart failure may arise as a result of various factors, such as:

- **Coronary Artery Disease (CAD):** The most common cause of heart failure.
- **High Blood Pressure:** Hypertension can lead to an enlarged heart and weakened muscle.
- **Heart Valve Disease:** Problems with heart valves can affect blood flow.
- **Cardiomyopathy:** Damage to the heart muscle.
- **Diabetes:** Uncontrolled diabetes can damage blood vessels and the heart.
- **Certain Medications:** Some medications can contribute to heart failure.
- **Overindulgence in Alcohol:** May cause the heart muscle to weaken.
- **Smoking:** Smoking is a risk factor for heart disease and heart failure.
- **Congenital Heart Defects:** Structural heart issues present at birth.
- **Infections:** Certain infections can affect the heart.

Symptoms:

Symptoms of heart failure can include:

 - Breathing difficulties, particularly when lying down or engaging in strenuous exercise.
- Fatigue and weakness.
- Swelling of the ankles, feet, and legs is known as edema.
- Rapid or irregular heartbeat.
- Persistent cough or wheezing.
- Increased need to urinate at night.

Diagnosis:

Diagnosing heart failure involves a combination of medical history, physical examination, and various tests, including echocardiograms, electrocardiograms (ECGs), and blood tests to measure specific markers.

Treatment:

The treatment of heart failure typically involves:

1. **Lifestyle Changes:** This includes dietary modifications to reduce salt intake, fluid restriction (in some cases), and regular physical activity under medical supervision.

2. **Medications:** Various drugs may be prescribed to control symptoms, improve heart function, and reduce the progression of the disease.

3. **Medical Procedures:** In some cases, procedures like coronary artery angioplasty, valve repair or replacement, and implantation of devices like pacemakers or defibrillators may be necessary.

4. **Heart Transplant:** For severe cases where other treatments are ineffective, heart transplantation may be considered.

Heart failure is a chronic condition that requires ongoing management and close medical monitoring. With proper care and adherence to treatment plans, individuals with heart failure can lead fulfilling lives and manage their symptoms effectively.

ARRHYTHMIAS

Arrhythmias:

Arrhythmias are irregular heart rhythms, which can manifest as heartbeats that are too fast (tachycardia), too slow (bradycardia), or irregular. These abnormalities can occur in the heart's electrical system, disrupting the heart's natural rhythm. Arrhythmias can range from harmless to life-threatening, and they may be temporary or persistent.

Types of Arrhythmias:

1. **Atrial Fibrillation (AFib):** AFib is one of the most common arrhythmias, characterized by rapid and irregular electrical signals in the heart's upper chambers (atria). It can lead to an increased risk of stroke and other heart-related complications.

2. **Atrial Flutter:** Similar to AFib, but the electrical signals are more organized and less chaotic.

3. **Ventricular Tachycardia:** This is a fast and potentially life-threatening rhythm that originates in the heart's lower chambers (ventricles).

4. **Ventricular Fibrillation:** A chaotic and life-threatening arrhythmia that causes the heart's ventricles to quiver instead of pumping blood effectively. It's a medical emergency.

5. **Bradycardia:** This is a slow heart rate, often defined as fewer than 60 beats per minute.

6. **Supraventricular Tachycardia (SVT):** SVT includes various rapid heart rhythms that originate above the ventricles.

7. **Premature Contractions:** These are early beats that disrupt the regular heart rhythm, including premature atrial contractions (PACs) and premature ventricular contractions (PVCs).

Causes and Risk Factors:

Arrhythmias may result from a number of causes, such as:

- Coronary artery disease (CAD)
- High blood pressure
- Heart attacks
- Heart valve disorders
- Congenital heart defects
- Diabetes

- Excessive alcohol or caffeine consumption
- Smoking
- Medications
- Stimulants
- Stress and anxiety
- Electrolyte imbalances

Symptoms:

Depending on the kind and degree of the ailment, arrhythmia symptoms can change. Common symptoms include:

- Palpitations (a fluttering or pounding in the chest)
- Dizziness or lightheadedness
- Fainting (syncope)
- Chest pain or discomfort
- Shortness of breath
- Fatigue

Diagnosis:

Arrhythmias can be diagnosed through various tests, including electrocardiograms (ECGs), Holter monitoring, event monitoring, and electrophysiology studies.

Treatment:

The kind and severity of an arrhythmia determine how it should be treated. It may include:

1. **Lifestyle Modifications:** Avoiding triggers like caffeine, alcohol, and stress.
2. **Medications:** Anti-arrhythmic drugs may be prescribed to control the heart's rhythm.
3. **Cardioversion:** Using electrical shocks or medications to restore a regular rhythm.
4. **Catheter Ablation:** A procedure to correct arrhythmias by destroying the abnormal heart tissue.
5. **Implantable Devices:** Pacemakers or implantable cardioverter-defibrillators (ICDs) can regulate the heart's rhythm and provide shock therapy if needed.

For life-threatening arrhythmias, immediate medical attention is necessary, and treatments like cardiopulmonary resuscitation (CPR) and defibrillation may be required.

It's important to consult with a healthcare professional for proper diagnosis and treatment of arrhythmias, as treatment plans vary depending on the specific type and severity of the condition.

VALVULAR HEART DISEASE

Valvular heart disease refers to conditions where the heart's valves, which control the flow of blood in and out of the heart's chambers, do not function properly. These conditions can affect the opening and closing of the heart valves, leading to problems with blood flow through the heart.

Types of Valvular Heart Disease:

There are several types of valvular heart disease, including:

1. **Aortic Stenosis:** This condition occurs when the aortic valve becomes narrowed or calcified, reducing blood flow from the left ventricle to the aorta.

2. **Aortic Regurgitation (Aortic Insufficiency):** In this condition, the aortic valve does not close properly, allowing blood to flow backward into the left ventricle.

3. **Mitral Stenosis:** Mitral stenosis involves a narrowing of the mitral valve, which separates the left atrium from the left ventricle.

4. **Mitral Regurgitation (Mitral Insufficiency):** In this condition, the mitral valve fails to close completely, allowing blood to flow backward from the left ventricle into the left atrium.

5. **Tricuspid Stenosis:** Tricuspid stenosis is characterized by a narrowing of the tricuspid valve, which separates the right atrium from the right ventricle.

6. **Tricuspid Regurgitation:** In this condition, the tricuspid valve does not close properly, leading to

blood flowing backward from the right ventricle into the right atrium.

Causes and Risk Factors:

Valvular heart disease can result from a variety of factors, including congenital heart defects, age-related changes, infections, rheumatic fever, and other underlying heart conditions.

Symptoms:

Valvular heart disease symptoms might differ according on the kind and degree of the illness. Common symptoms include:

- Fatigue
- Breathlessness, particularly when exerted physically
- Palpitations (irregular heartbeats)
- Chest pain or discomfort
- Edema, or ankle and foot swelling
- Fainting (syncope)

Diagnosis:

Diagnosis of valvular heart disease involves a combination of medical history, physical examination, and various tests, such as echocardiograms, electrocardiograms (ECGs), and cardiac catheterization.

Treatment:

The treatment of valvular heart disease depends on the type and severity of the condition. Options may include:

1. **Medications:** Medications can help manage symptoms and prevent complications, such as blood pressure control and anticoagulants to reduce the risk of blood clots.

2. **Valvuloplasty:** In some cases, a minimally invasive procedure may be performed to repair or widen a narrowed valve.

3. **Valve Repair or Replacement:** Severe valve disease may require surgical repair or replacement of the affected valve with either a mechanical or biological valve.

4. **Transcatheter Valve Replacement:** A less invasive option for valve replacement, typically used for high-risk patients.

The choice of treatment depends on factors such as the type of valve affected, the severity of the condition, the patient's overall health, and individual preferences. Valvular heart disease management often involves a multidisciplinary team, including cardiologists and cardiac surgeons.

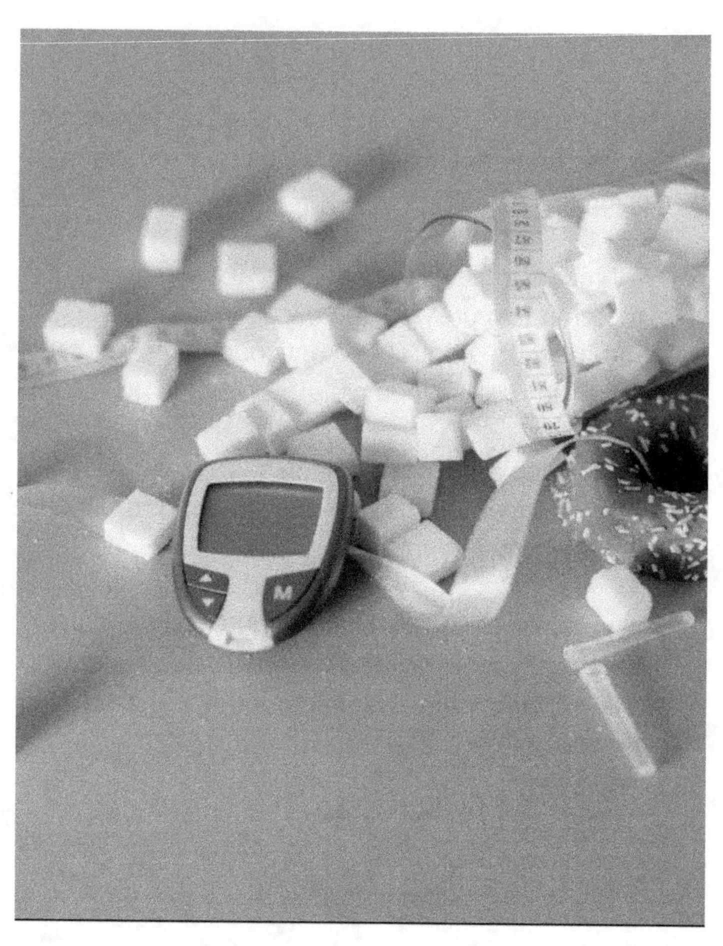

CHAPTER THREE

RISK FACTORS AND HEART HEALTH

Understanding the risk factors associated with heart disease is crucial for prevention and early intervention. Some risk factors can be modified through lifestyle changes, while others are non-modifiable. Here are some of the key risk factors for heart health:

Modifiable Risk Factors:

1. **High Blood Pressure (Hypertension):** Elevated blood pressure can damage the arteries, making them more susceptible to plaque buildup. Lifestyle changes and medications can help control blood pressure.

2. **High Cholesterol:** High levels of low-density lipoprotein (LDL) cholesterol can lead to the buildup of plaque in the arteries. A heart-healthy diet, regular exercise, and medications can help manage cholesterol levels.

3. **Smoking:** Tobacco use is a major risk factor for heart disease. Quitting smoking significantly reduces the risk.

4. **Unhealthy Diet:** Diets high in saturated and trans fats, sodium, and added sugars can contribute to heart disease. It is advised to eat a diet high in fruits, vegetables, whole grains, and lean meats.

5. **Physical Inactivity:** A sedentary lifestyle can lead to obesity, high blood pressure, and other risk factors. Getting regular exercise is crucial for heart health.

6. **Obesity:** Excess body weight increases the risk of heart disease, particularly if the weight is centered around the abdomen.

7. **Diabetes:** High blood sugar levels can damage blood vessels and increase the risk of heart disease. For heart health, diabetes management is essential.

8. **Excessive Alcohol Consumption:** Heavy drinking can lead to high blood pressure, heart muscle damage, and irregular heart rhythms. Moderation is key.

9. **Stress:** Chronic stress can contribute to heart disease. Exercise and stress reduction methods like meditation can be beneficial.

10. **Sleep Apnea:** This condition, which causes interrupted breathing during sleep, is associated with an increased risk of heart disease.

Non-Modifiable Risk Factors:

1. **Age:** The risk of heart disease increases with age, especially for individuals over 65.

2. **Gender:** Men are generally at a higher risk of heart disease; however, the risk for women increases after menopause.

3. **Family History:** A family history of heart disease can raise an individual's risk.

4. **Genetics:** Certain genetic factors can predispose individuals to heart disease.

5. **Race and Ethnicity:** Some racial and ethnic groups are at a higher risk of heart disease.

Other Risk Factors:

1. **High Levels of Inflammation:** Chronic inflammation in the body is associated with an increased risk of heart disease.

2. **Illegal Drug Use:** The use of illegal drugs, such as cocaine and amphetamines, can lead to heart-related issues.

3. **Environmental Factors:** Air pollution and exposure to toxins can contribute to heart disease risk.

It's important to note that these risk factors can often interact with each other, compounding the risk. For example, obesity can lead to high blood pressure and diabetes. Addressing modifiable risk factors through lifestyle changes and, when necessary, medical management, can significantly reduce the risk of heart disease. Regular check-ups with healthcare professionals are essential to monitor and manage these risk factors.

THE INTERPLAY OF GENETICS AND LIFESTYLE

Heart health is influenced by a complex interplay between genetics and lifestyle factors. Understanding how these two elements interact is essential in assessing an individual's risk for heart disease and in tailoring strategies for prevention and management.

Genetics:

The risk of heart disease in an individual is influenced by genetic variables. Some people may inherit genes that make them more prone to specific risk factors, such as high cholesterol or high blood pressure. Key aspects of the genetic influence on heart health include:

1. **Family History:** A family history of heart disease can be a strong indicator of genetic risk. If close relatives have had heart disease, heart attacks, or other related conditions, your risk may be elevated.

2. **Genetic Variants:** Specific genetic variations can increase the risk of heart disease. For example, there are genes associated with elevated cholesterol levels or blood clotting disorders.

3. **Polygenic Risk:** Heart disease is often influenced by multiple genes, each contributing in a small way. A polygenic risk score can assess an individual's overall genetic susceptibility.

Lifestyle Factors:

Lifestyle plays a significant role in heart health, and many risk factors for heart disease are influenced by individual choices and behaviors. Lifestyle factors that affect heart health include:

1. **Diet:** An unhealthy diet high in saturated fats, trans fats, sodium, and added sugars can contribute to heart disease. Conversely, a heart-healthy diet rich in fruits, vegetables, whole grains, and lean proteins can lower the risk.

2. **Physical Activity:** Regular exercise can help maintain a healthy weight, reduce high blood

pressure, and improve cholesterol levels, all of which promote heart health.

3. **Smoking:** Tobacco use is a major risk factor for heart disease. Quitting smoking is one of the most effective ways to reduce heart disease risk.

4. **Alcohol Consumption:** Excessive alcohol intake can lead to high blood pressure and other heart-related issues. Moderation is recommended.

5. **Stress Management:** Chronic stress can contribute to heart disease. This risk can be reduced with the aid of efficient stress management strategies.

6. **Weight Management:** Maintaining a healthy weight is crucial for heart health. Obesity is a significant risk factor.

The Interplay:

The interplay between genetics and lifestyle is complex. While genetics can influence an individual's baseline risk for heart disease, lifestyle factors can modify and exacerbate that risk. For example:

- A person with a genetic predisposition for high cholesterol can further increase their risk by consuming an unhealthy diet high in saturated fats.

- Genetics may contribute to an increased likelihood of high blood pressure, but regular exercise and a low-sodium diet can help manage it.

Understanding this interplay is essential for personalized heart disease prevention and management. Those with a strong family history or genetic risk factors should pay close attention to their lifestyle choices, focusing on a heart-healthy diet, regular exercise, and other lifestyle modifications to lower their overall risk. Healthcare professionals can provide guidance and recommend appropriate screenings or genetic tests when necessary.

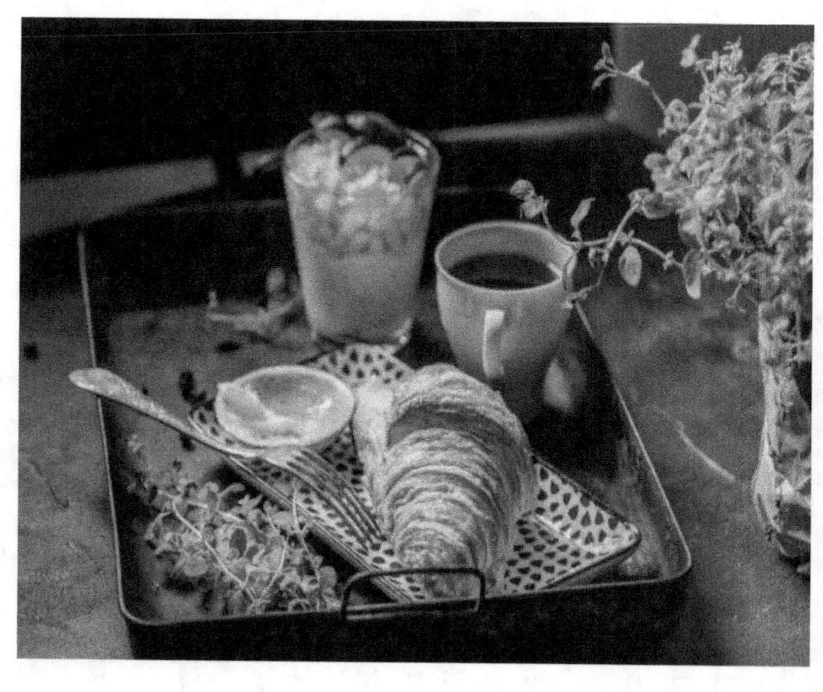

CHAPTER FOUR

THE HEART-HEALTHY DIET

A heart-healthy diet is a crucial component of maintaining and improving cardiovascular health. It focuses on making dietary choices that promote heart health, reduce the risk of heart disease, and manage existing heart conditions. Here are the key principles of a heart-healthy diet:

1. **Limit Saturated and Trans Fats:**
   - Reduce the consumption of saturated fats found in red meat, full-fat dairy products, and tropical oils like coconut and palm oil.
   - Steer clear of trans fats, which are frequently included in fried and processed foods. Check food labels for the term "partially hydrogenated oils."

2. **Choose Heart-Healthy Fats:**
   - Opt for unsaturated fats, such as those found in olive oil, canola oil, avocados, and nuts. These fats can lower the risk of heart disease and help raise cholesterol levels.

3. **Consume Omega-3 Fatty Acids:**
   - Include sources of omega-3 fatty acids in your diet, like fatty fish (salmon, mackerel, trout), flaxseeds, and walnuts. Omega-3s are known for their heart-protective properties.

4. **Increase Fiber Intake:**
   - Eat a variety of fiber-rich foods like whole grains, fruits, vegetables, legumes, and nuts. Fiber lowers cholesterol, which is beneficial to heart health.

5. **Control Portion Sizes:**
   - Pay attention to portion sizes in order to avoid overindulging and to keep a healthy weight. In order to reduce calorie consumption, portion control is essential.

6. **Limit Sodium (Salt) Intake:**
   - Reduce the consumption of high-sodium foods, such as processed and fast foods. Instead of using a lot of salt to flavor your food, use herbs and spices.

7. **Choose Lean Proteins:**
   - Opt for lean protein sources like skinless poultry, fish, legumes, and lean cuts of meat. Consume as little red meat as possible, especially processed meats.

8. **Include Fruits and Vegetables:**
   - Aim to fill half your plate with a variety of colorful fruits and vegetables. They are rich in vitamins, minerals, and antioxidants that support heart health.

9. **Watch Sugar Intake:**

- Limit added sugars in your diet. Sugary beverages, sweets, and sugary cereals should be consumed in moderation.

10. **Control Alcohol Consumption:**
   - If you consume alcohol, do it sparingly. For women, this means up to one drink per day; for men, up to two drinks per day.

11. **Stay Hydrated:**
   - Drink plenty of water and consider replacing sugary drinks with water, herbal tea, or unsweetened beverages.

12. **Meal Planning and Preparation:**
   - Arrange your meals in advance to choose better options. You have control over the ingredients and portion quantities when you cook at home.

13. **Limit Processed Foods:**
   - Minimize processed and fast foods, as they often contain unhealthy fats, high levels of sodium, and hidden additives.

14. **Mindful Eating:**
   - Eat mindfully by being aware of your body's signals of hunger and fullness. Steer clear of eating while preoccupied or in front of screens.

15. **Regular Eating Schedule:**
   - Aim for regular meal times to stabilize blood sugar levels and control hunger.

Remember that a heart-healthy diet is not a one-size-fits-all approach. It's essential to personalize your diet to your specific health needs and preferences. If you have specific dietary concerns or conditions, such as diabetes or high cholesterol, consult with a healthcare professional or registered dietitian to create a tailored heart-healthy eating plan. Additionally, combining a heart-healthy diet with regular physical activity and other heart-protective lifestyle habits can provide comprehensive support for your cardiovascular health.

FOOD TO INCLUDE

To maintain a heart-healthy diet, include a variety of foods that offer cardiovascular benefits. The following foods ought to be a part of your diet:

1. **Fruits:** Incorporate a wide range of fruits such as berries, citrus fruits, apples, and pears. They are rich in vitamins, minerals, and antioxidants that support heart health.

2. **Vegetables:** Consume a colorful assortment of vegetables, including leafy greens, broccoli, carrots, and bell peppers. These provide fiber and essential nutrients.

3. **Whole Grains:** Choose whole grains like oats, brown rice, whole wheat pasta, and quinoa. They are high in fiber and can help lower cholesterol levels.

4. **Fatty Fish:** Include fatty fish like salmon, mackerel, sardines, and trout in your diet. They are excellent sources of heart-protective omega-3 fatty acids.

5. **Nuts and Seeds:** Snack on unsalted nuts such as almonds, walnuts, and pistachios. Add flaxseeds, chia seeds, and sunflower seeds to your meals for added healthy fats and fiber.

6. **Legumes:** Incorporate beans, lentils, chickpeas, and peas into soups, salads, and stews. Both fiber and plant-based protein are abundant in them.

7. **Lean Proteins:** Opt for lean protein sources like skinless poultry, turkey, and tofu. Saturated fat content is lower in these selections.

8. **Olive Oil:** Use extra virgin olive oil for cooking and in salad dressings. It's a source of monounsaturated fats that can benefit heart health.

9. **Avocados:** Enjoy avocados in salads, sandwiches, or as a spread. They include plenty of healthy fats and fiber.

10. **Low-Fat Dairy or Dairy Alternatives:** If you consume dairy, choose low-fat or fat-free options. Dairy alternatives like almond milk or soy milk are also heart-healthy choices.

11. **Berries:** Berries like blueberries, strawberries, and raspberries are packed with antioxidants and can help reduce inflammation.

12. **Tomatoes:** Tomatoes are a good source of lycopene, an antioxidant linked to heart health. Cooked tomato products like tomato sauce and tomato paste can be particularly beneficial.

13. **Garlic:** Garlic has potential cardiovascular benefits and can be used to add flavor to dishes.

14. **Green Tea:** Green tea contains antioxidants that may contribute to heart health. It can be a healthy alternative to sugary or caffeinated beverages.

15. **Dark Chocolate (in moderation):** Dark chocolate with a high cocoa content (70% or more) may have heart-healthy properties. Enjoy it in moderation.

16. **Herbs and Spices:** Season your dishes with herbs and spices like oregano, basil, and cinnamon, which can add flavor without excessive salt or sugar.

17. **Flaxseeds:** Sprinkle ground flaxseeds on cereals or yogurt. They are rich in fiber, omega-3 fatty acids, and lignans, which may benefit heart health.

18. **Turmeric:** Turmeric contains curcumin, which has anti-inflammatory properties. It can be added to food or used in cooking.

Incorporating these foods into your diet while following a balanced and heart-healthy eating plan can help support your cardiovascular health and reduce the risk of heart disease. Remember that portion control and overall dietary patterns are equally important in maintaining a heart-healthy lifestyle.

FOOD TO AVOID

To maintain a heart-healthy diet and reduce the risk of heart disease, it's important to limit or avoid certain foods that are high in unhealthy fats, added sugars, and sodium. The following foods ought to be consumed in moderation or should be avoided:

1. **Saturated and Trans Fats:** Limit foods high in saturated and trans fats, as they can raise cholesterol levels and increase the risk of heart disease. Avoid or minimize:

   - Red meat, especially fatty cuts

- processed meats, including hot dogs
- Full-fat dairy products
- Palm and coconut oil
- Commercially baked goods with hydrogenated or partially hydrogenated oils

2. **High-Sodium Foods:** Excessive sodium intake can lead to high blood pressure, a significant risk factor for heart disease. Avoid or reduce:

- Processed and packaged foods (canned soups, frozen meals, processed snacks)
- Fast food and restaurant fare (which is frequently sodium-rich)
- Excessive use of table salt
- High-sodium condiments like soy sauce and salad dressings

3. **Added Sugars:** High sugar consumption can contribute to weight gain and increase the risk of heart disease. Limit or avoid:

- Sugary drinks, such as energy drinks, fruit juices, and sodas
- Candy, sugary snacks, and desserts
- Foods with added sugars in the ingredients list (check labels)

4. **Trans Fats:** Trans fats are particularly harmful to heart health. They may cause levels of LDL (bad) and HDL (good) cholesterol to rise and fall, respectively. Avoid foods with partially

hydrogenated oils, which often contain trans fats. These may include:

  - Many commercially baked goods (cakes, cookies, doughnuts)
    - Fried foods (some fast-food items)
    - Some margarines and vegetable shortening

5. **Excess Alcohol:** While moderate alcohol consumption may have some heart-protective effects, excessive drinking can lead to high blood pressure and other heart-related issues. If you do drink, limit your intake to no more than one drink for women and two for men per day.

6. **Processed and Fast Foods:** These often contain unhealthy fats, excessive sodium, and hidden additives. Reducing the intake of processed and fast foods can significantly improve heart health.

7. **Highly Processed Snacks:** Snack foods like chips, crackers, and store-bought pastries tend to be high in unhealthy fats, sodium, and often contain added sugars.

8. **Fried Foods:** Fried foods, such as deep-fried chicken, french fries, and other fried snacks, are often high in unhealthy fats and calories.

9. **Sugary Cereals:** Many breakfast cereals marketed to children can be high in added sugars. Choose cereals with lower sugar content.

10. **Highly Sweetened and Sugary Breakfast Pastries:** Items like sweet rolls and sugary muffins can be high in added sugars and unhealthy fats.

It's critical to read food labels and be informed about the components of the goods you buy. To maintain a heart-healthy diet, focus on fresh, whole foods, and prepare meals at home whenever possible. Reducing the consumption of foods high in unhealthy fats, added sugars, and sodium while increasing the intake of fruits, vegetables, whole grains, and lean proteins can have a positive impact on your heart health.

PORTION CONTROL AND BALANCED EATING

Portion control and balanced eating are essential components of a heart-healthy diet. They help you manage calorie intake, maintain a healthy weight, and ensure you get a variety of nutrients to support your cardiovascular health. Here's how to practice portion control and balanced eating:

Portion Control:

1. **Be Mindful of Serving Sizes:** Learn to recognize appropriate portion sizes for different

types of foods. Use measuring cups and a kitchen scale if needed to become familiar with recommended serving sizes.

2. **Use Smaller Plates:** Opt for smaller plates and bowls to help control portion sizes. A smaller plate can make a moderate portion of food appear satisfying.

3. **Avoid "Supersizing":** Be cautious of large portions at restaurants and fast-food establishments. Choose smaller sizes or share larger meals when dining out.

4. **Practice the Plate Method:** When preparing meals, envision your plate divided into sections:
   - Vegetables and fruits should account for half of your plate.
   - Allocate one-quarter of your plate to lean protein.
   - Keep the remaining 1/4 for vegetables or whole grains.

5. **Listen to Your Body:** Observe the signals your body sends when it is hungry or full. Eat only when it's necessary and stop when you're satisfied.

6. **Limit Buffets and All-You-Can-Eat Settings:** These environments can encourage overeating. If you find yourself at a buffet, choose smaller portions and make healthier choices.

Balanced Eating:

1. **Incorporate All Food Groups:** Ensure your meals include foods from all food groups: fruits, vegetables, lean proteins, whole grains, and healthy fats. This balance provides a wide range of nutrients.

2. **Choose Whole Foods:** Focus on whole, unprocessed foods. These are often more nutritious and contain fewer unhealthy additives.

3. **Prioritize Fiber:** Include fiber-rich foods like whole grains, legumes, fruits, and vegetables. Fiber promotes fullness and supports heart health.

4. **Healthy Fats:** Include foods like avocados, almonds, seeds, and olive oil that are good sources of fat. These fats can improve cholesterol levels.

5. **Lean Proteins:** Select lean protein sources, including skinless poultry, fish, tofu, and legumes. Limit red and processed meats.

6. **Colorful Fruits and Vegetables:** Aim for a variety of colorful fruits and vegetables, as different colors often indicate a diverse range of nutrients and antioxidants.

7. **Limit Added Sugars:** Minimize foods and beverages with added sugars. Opt for naturally sweet options like whole fruits.

8. **Moderate Salt Intake:** Be conscious of sodium content in your food. Limit high-sodium condiments and processed foods.

9. **Stay Hydrated:** Throughout the day, sip a lot of water. Sometimes thirst is mistaken for hunger.

10. **Plan Balanced Meals:** When preparing meals, aim to create a balanced plate with a mix of foods from different food groups.

11. **Regular Meal Schedule:** Establish regular meal times and avoid skipping meals. Eating at consistent intervals helps stabilize blood sugar levels.

12. **Cook at Home:** Preparing meals at home gives you control over ingredients and portion sizes. It allows you to make healthier choices.

Remember that balanced eating doesn't mean you have to eliminate all indulgent or less nutritious foods. The key is moderation. It's perfectly fine to enjoy occasional treats, as long as they don't dominate your regular diet.

Balanced eating and portion control work together to help you maintain a heart-healthy diet and reduce the risk of heart disease. Consistently practicing these habits can lead to better heart health and overall well-being.

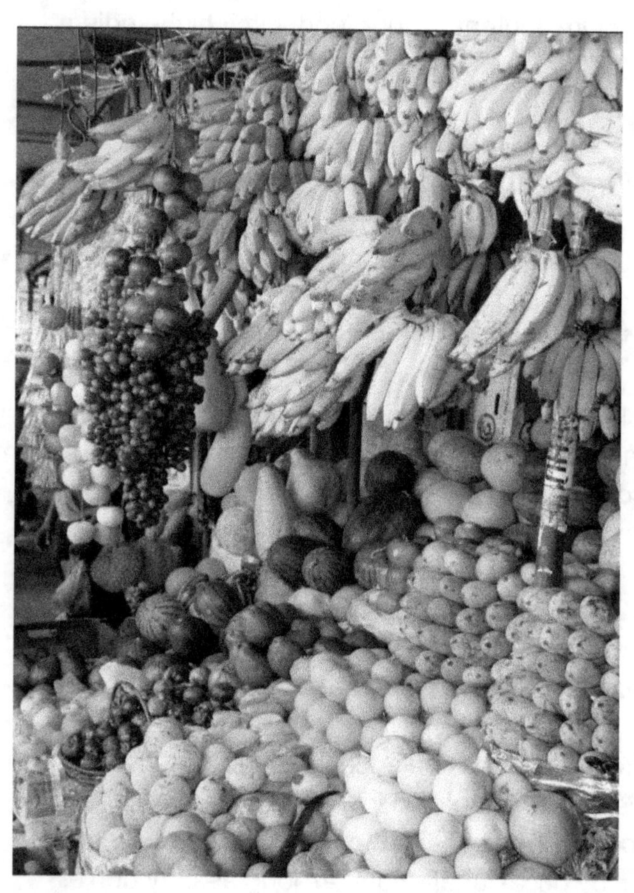

CHAPTER FIVE

UNDERSTANDING CHOLESTEROL

Cholesterol is a type of fat (lipid) that is essential for the proper functioning of your body. It is a crucial component of cell membranes, aids in the production of hormones, and is involved in the digestion of dietary fats. Cholesterol is produced by your liver and is also obtained from the food you eat. To understand cholesterol better, let's break down some key aspects:

Types of Cholesterol:

1. **Low-Density Lipoprotein (LDL) Cholesterol:** Often referred to as "bad" cholesterol, LDL cholesterol carries cholesterol particles from the liver to cells throughout the body. When there is an excess of LDL cholesterol, it can lead to the buildup of fatty deposits in the arteries, contributing to atherosclerosis (plaque formation) and an increased risk of heart disease.

2. **High-Density Lipoprotein (HDL) Cholesterol:** Known as "good" cholesterol, HDL cholesterol has the role of transporting excess cholesterol from the bloodstream back to the liver for excretion. High

levels of HDL cholesterol are associated with a lower risk of heart disease.

Total Cholesterol: This value represents the combined levels of both LDL and HDL cholesterol in your blood.

Triglycerides: Triglycerides are a type of fat found in your blood, and high levels of triglycerides can also increase the risk of heart disease, particularly when combined with high LDL cholesterol.

Cholesterol Levels:

Healthy cholesterol levels are essential for cardiovascular health. Ideal cholesterol levels can vary depending on your overall health and medical history, but in general, lower LDL cholesterol and higher HDL cholesterol are desirable. Elevated LDL cholesterol levels are a risk factor for atherosclerosis and heart disease.

Cholesterol Sources:

Cholesterol comes from two primary sources:

1. **Dietary Cholesterol:** You obtain dietary cholesterol from animal-based foods such as meat, poultry, fish, eggs, and dairy products. However, dietary cholesterol has a smaller impact on your blood cholesterol levels than was once thought. For

many people, saturated and trans fats in the diet have a more significant influence on LDL cholesterol levels.

2. **Liver Production:** Your liver naturally produces cholesterol to meet the body's requirements. The liver's production of cholesterol is influenced by genetics and dietary intake.

Cholesterol and Heart Health:

Elevated LDL cholesterol levels are a significant risk factor for atherosclerosis, which can lead to heart attacks and strokes. Reducing LDL cholesterol through lifestyle changes (e.g., dietary modifications, exercise) and, when necessary, medication can help lower this risk.

Maintaining or increasing HDL cholesterol levels is associated with a reduced risk of heart disease because HDL helps clear excess cholesterol from the bloodstream.

Cholesterol Testing:

A lipid panel blood test can be used to determine cholesterol levels. This test provides information about your LDL, HDL, and total cholesterol levels, as well as triglycerides.

Cholesterol Management:

Controlling your cholesterol levels is critical for good heart health. Lifestyle changes, including a heart-healthy diet, regular exercise, and avoiding smoking, are effective ways to control cholesterol. In some cases, healthcare providers may prescribe medications, such as statins, to help lower LDL cholesterol.

Understanding your cholesterol levels and making the necessary adjustments to your lifestyle and, if needed, medications can significantly reduce the risk of heart disease and improve your overall cardiovascular health. It's important to work with a healthcare professional to determine the most appropriate approach for your specific situation.

DIETARY STRATEGIES FOR LOWERING LDL CHOLESTEROL

Lowering LDL (low-density lipoprotein) cholesterol through dietary strategies is a key component of heart disease prevention and management. High LDL cholesterol levels are associated with an increased risk of atherosclerosis and heart disease. Here are dietary strategies to help lower LDL cholesterol:

1. **Choose Heart-Healthy Fats:**
   - Choose monounsaturated fats (found in olive oil, avocados, and almonds) and polyunsaturated fats

(found in fatty fish, flaxseeds, and walnuts). These lipids may aid in the reduction of LDL cholesterol.

2. **Limit Saturated Fats:**
   - Reduce your intake of saturated fats, which are often found in red meat, full-fat dairy products, and tropical oils like coconut and palm oil. These lipids have the potential to elevate LDL cholesterol levels.

3. **Avoid Trans Fats:**
   - Completely eliminate trans fats from your diet. Trans fats are often found in processed and fried foods. Examine food labels for the phrase "partially hydrogenated oils."

4. **Consume More Soluble Fiber:**
   - Foods rich in soluble fiber, such as oats, barley, beans, lentils, fruits, and vegetables, can help lower LDL cholesterol levels. Make an effort to consume at least 5-10 grams of soluble fiber every day.

5. **Include Plant Sterols and Stanols:**
   - Some margarines, spreads, and fortified foods contain plant sterols and stanols, which can help lower LDL cholesterol when consumed as part of a heart-healthy diet.

6. **Choose Whole Grains:**
   - Replace refined grains with whole grains like whole wheat, oats, brown rice, and quinoa. Whole grains are a good source of dietary fiber, which can help lower cholesterol.

7. **Eat Fatty Fish:**
   - Include fatty fish in your diet, such as salmon, mackerel, sardines, and trout. These fish are rich in omega-3 fatty acids, which have heart-protective properties.

8. **Nuts and Seeds:**
   - Snack on unsalted nuts such as almonds, walnuts, and pistachios. Add flaxseeds, chia seeds, and sunflower seeds to your meals for their healthy fats and fiber.

9. **Limit Red Meat and Processed Meats:**
   - Reduce the consumption of red meat, particularly fatty cuts. Minimize processed meats like sausages and bacon, which are high in saturated fats.

10. **Use Olive Oil:**
   - Cook with extra virgin olive oil, which is a source of heart-healthy monounsaturated fats.

11. **Increase Fruits and Vegetables:**
   - Aim to fill half your plate with a variety of colorful fruits and vegetables. Fiber, vitamins, minerals, and antioxidants are abundant in these foods.

12. **Garlic and Onions:**

- Include garlic and onions in your recipes. These ingredients may have a mild cholesterol-lowering effect.

13. **Tea:**
   - Consider drinking black or green tea, which contains compounds called catechins that may help lower LDL cholesterol.

14. **Limit Added Sugars:**
   - Minimize foods and beverages with added sugars, as excessive sugar intake can contribute to heart disease risk.

15. **Moderate Alcohol Consumption:**
- Drink in moderation if you consume alcohol. For women, this means up to one drink per day; for men, up to two drinks per day.

16. **Portion Control:**
   - Be mindful of portion sizes to avoid overeating and manage calorie Intake, which can impact cholesterol levels.

It's important to note that the effectiveness of dietary strategies may vary from person to person. Before making significant dietary changes to lower LDL cholesterol, consult with a healthcare professional or a registered dietitian to create a personalized plan that considers your specific health needs and dietary preferences. Additionally, combining dietary modifications with regular physical activity and, if necessary, prescribed medications can provide comprehensive support for managing cholesterol and improving heart health.

THE IMPORTANCE OF HDL CHOLESTEROL

High-Density Lipoprotein (HDL) cholesterol is often referred to as "good" cholesterol, and it plays a crucial role in maintaining cardiovascular health. While you may be more familiar with the emphasis on reducing "bad" LDL (Low-Density Lipoprotein) cholesterol levels, understanding the importance of HDL cholesterol is equally essential. Here's why HDL cholesterol is significant for your overall health:

1. **Heart Disease Protection:** One of the primary functions of HDL cholesterol is to transport excess cholesterol from the bloodstream to the liver for disposal. This process helps prevent the buildup of cholesterol in the arteries, which can lead to atherosclerosis (narrowing and hardening of the arteries) and an increased risk of heart disease.

2. **Atherosclerosis Prevention:** HDL cholesterol acts as a scavenger in the bloodstream, collecting cholesterol deposited in the arterial walls and returning it to the liver. This protective mechanism helps keep your arteries clear of plaque, reducing the risk of blockages and cardiovascular events.

3. **Anti-Inflammatory Properties:** HDL cholesterol has anti-inflammatory effects, which can help reduce the inflammation that contributes to atherosclerosis and other heart-related conditions.

4. **Blood Clot Prevention:** HDL cholesterol can inhibit blood clot formation by reducing the stickiness of platelets in the blood, further decreasing the risk of heart attacks and strokes.

5. **Antioxidant Activity:** HDL cholesterol has antioxidant properties, which means it can help protect the body's cells and tissues from oxidative damage, including the oxidative damage that occurs in the arteries.

6. **Reverse Cholesterol Transport:** HDL cholesterol participates in a process known as "reverse cholesterol transport," in which it removes excess cholesterol from cells and tissues, helping to maintain a healthy cholesterol balance throughout the body.

HDL Cholesterol Levels:

Ideally, you want higher levels of HDL cholesterol in your bloodstream, as they are associated with a reduced risk of heart disease. A higher HDL cholesterol level is generally considered protective. Conversely, low levels of HDL cholesterol can increase the risk of heart disease, even if your LDL cholesterol levels are within a healthy range.

Factors That Can Raise HDL Cholesterol:

Several lifestyle factors and habits can help raise HDL cholesterol levels, including:

- Regular physical activity: Exercise, particularly aerobic activities like brisk walking, running, and swimming, can increase HDL cholesterol.
- Consuming healthy fats: Replacing saturated and trans fats in your diet with unsaturated fats, such as those found in olive oil and fatty fish, can positively impact HDL cholesterol.
- Moderate alcohol consumption: For some individuals, moderate alcohol intake (up to one drink per day for women and up to two drinks per day for men) can lead to increased HDL cholesterol. However, alcohol should be consumed in moderation and is not recommended for everyone.

In Conclusion:

Understanding the importance of HDL cholesterol is essential for heart health. Having higher levels of HDL cholesterol can contribute to a lower risk of heart disease by promoting the removal of excess cholesterol from the arteries and providing other protective effects. To maintain or increase HDL cholesterol levels, adopt a heart-healthy lifestyle that includes regular exercise, a balanced diet, and other habits that support cardiovascular well-being.

It's also a good idea to consult with a healthcare professional to assess your cholesterol levels and receive personalized guidance on optimizing your heart health.

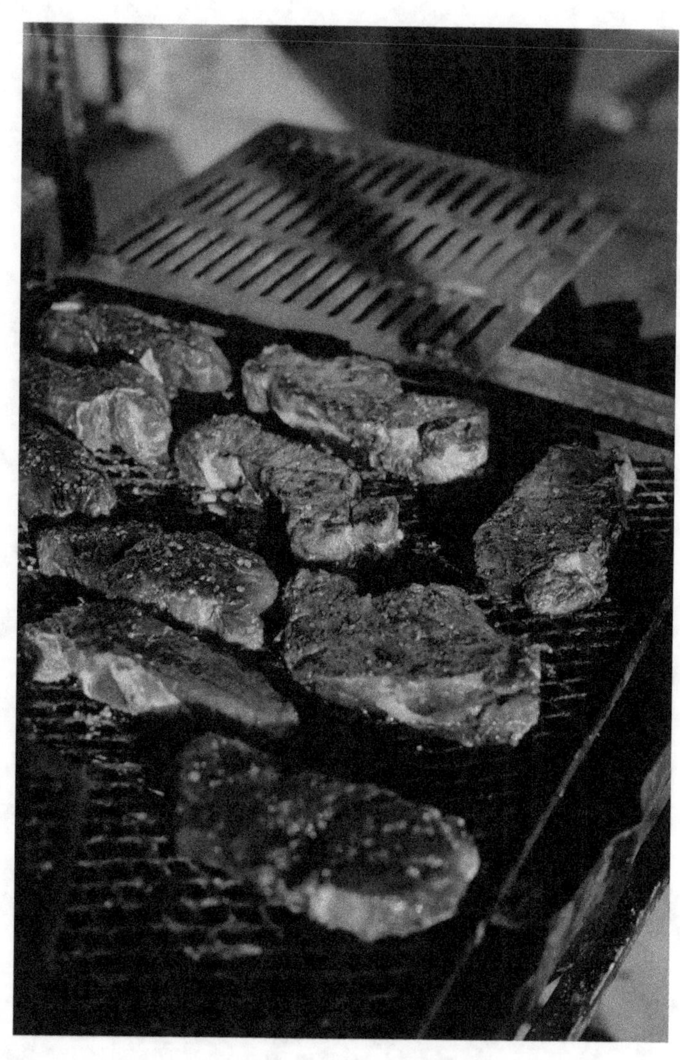

CHAPTER SIX

BLOOD PRESSURE AND DIETS

Blood pressure is a critical factor in cardiovascular health, and dietary choices can significantly impact blood pressure levels. High blood pressure (hypertension) is a major risk factor for heart disease, stroke, and other health conditions. Here are some dietary strategies to help manage and lower blood pressure:

1. DASH Diet: The Dietary Approaches to Stop Hypertension (DASH) diet is specifically designed to lower blood pressure. It emphasizes the following:

  - **Fruits and Vegetables:** Consume a variety of fruits and vegetables daily, which are rich in potassium, fiber, and antioxidants.
  - **Whole Grains:** Choose whole grains like brown rice, whole wheat bread, and oats for their fiber and nutrients.
  - **Lean Protein:** Opt for lean protein sources, such as skinless poultry, fish, and legumes, to reduce saturated fat intake.
  - **Nuts and Seeds:** Incorporate unsalted nuts and seeds for their heart-healthy fats, fiber, and magnesium.

   - **Dairy or Dairy Alternatives:** Include low-fat or fat-free dairy products to ensure adequate calcium intake.
   - **Limit Sodium (Salt):** Reduce high-sodium foods, and use herbs and spices for flavor instead of excessive salt.

2. Reduce Sodium Intake: Excess sodium can raise blood pressure. To reduce sodium in your diet:

   - Limit your intake of processed and quick foods, which are generally rich in salt.
   - Read food labels and select items with lower salt content.
   - Cook at home, allowing you to control the amount of salt in your meals.

3. Increase Potassium: Potassium helps balance sodium in the body and can have a beneficial effect on blood pressure. Potassium-rich foods include bananas, oranges, potatoes, sweet potatoes, spinach, and beans.

4. Magnesium: Magnesium is another mineral that can help regulate blood pressure. It's found in foods like nuts, seeds, whole grains, and leafy green vegetables.

5. Omega-3 Fatty Acids: Fatty fish, such as salmon, mackerel, and trout, are rich in omega-3 fatty acids, which can support heart health and help lower blood pressure.

6. Limit Alcohol: Excessive alcohol consumption can raise blood pressure.Consume alcohol in moderation.

7. Weight Management: Maintaining a healthy weight is essential for blood pressure control. Weight loss, if needed, can have a positive impact on blood pressure.

8. Limit Added Sugars: Reducing foods and beverages high in added sugars can help with weight management and blood pressure control.

9. Control Caffeine: For some individuals, excessive caffeine intake can temporarily raise blood pressure. Be mindful of your caffeine consumption and its effects on your blood pressure.

10. Calcium: Adequate calcium intake, primarily from low-fat dairy or fortified dairy alternatives, is important for overall heart health.

11. Monitor Blood Pressure: Regularly check your blood pressure and consult with a healthcare professional for guidance and management, especially if you have hypertension.

It's important to note that dietary changes may take time to have an effect on blood pressure, and individual responses can vary. A combination of dietary modifications, physical activity, stress management, and, if necessary, medications under the guidance of a healthcare professional can help manage and lower blood pressure effectively.

HYPERTENSION AND HEART DISEASE

High blood pressure, or hypertension, is a key risk factor for cardiovascular disease. Understanding the connection between hypertension and heart disease is essential for maintaining cardiovascular health. Here are key points to consider:

1. Hypertension as a Silent Risk Factor:

- Hypertension often goes unnoticed because it rarely causes symptoms in its early stages. This is why it's often referred to as a "silent killer." Many people are unaware they have high blood pressure until it is diagnosed through a routine check-up or until they experience complications.

2. Impact on the Cardiovascular System:

- Over time, high blood pressure can damage the blood vessels and the heart. The increased pressure on the arteries can lead to atherosclerosis (plaque buildup), making it harder for blood to flow through the vessels. This can result in narrowed or blocked arteries, which can lead to heart disease.

3. Increased Risk of Heart Disease:

- Hypertension is a significant risk factor for heart disease, including conditions like coronary artery disease (narrowing of the heart's blood vessels), heart attacks, heart failure, and arrhythmias (irregular heart rhythms). High blood pressure can directly contribute to these cardiovascular issues.

4. Role in Atherosclerosis:

- Hypertension can accelerate the development of atherosclerosis. The force of blood against the arterial walls can damage them, leading to inflammation and the deposition of cholesterol and other substances. This contributes to the formation of plaque in the arteries.

5. Impact on the Heart Muscle:

- The heart works harder when blood pressure is elevated, leading to an increase in the size of the heart's muscular walls. This can result in hypertrophy, which is the thickening of the heart muscle. This can weaken the heart and lead to heart failure over time.

6. Concomitant Risk Factors:

- Hypertension often coexists with other cardiovascular risk factors such as high cholesterol, diabetes, and obesity, which further increase the risk of heart disease.

7. Importance of Blood Pressure Control:

- Controlling hypertension is a crucial step in preventing heart disease. Lifestyle modifications, including dietary changes, regular physical activity, stress management, and weight control, can help lower blood pressure. In some cases, medication may be prescribed by a healthcare professional to manage hypertension.

8. Regular Monitoring:

- Regular blood pressure monitoring is essential, even if you don't have a history of hypertension. It's important to catch and manage high blood pressure early to reduce its impact on the heart and overall health.

9. Lifestyle Changes:

- Making heart-healthy lifestyle changes, such as adopting a balanced diet, increasing physical activity, quitting smoking, and reducing stress, can have a significant positive impact on blood pressure and heart health.

10. Consultation with Healthcare Professionals:

- If you have hypertension or are at risk due to family history or other factors, it's essential to consult with a healthcare professional. They can provide personalized guidance and recommend appropriate interventions to manage blood pressure and reduce the risk of heart disease.

In conclusion, hypertension is a major risk factor for heart disease, and its impact on the cardiovascular system is substantial. Managing blood pressure through lifestyle changes and, when necessary, medication, is essential for preventing heart disease and maintaining overall cardiovascular health. Regular check-ups and consultation with healthcare professionals are key components of hypertension and heart disease prevention.

SODIUM INTAKE AND BLOOD PRESSURE CONTROL

Reducing sodium intake is a critical component of blood pressure control and overall heart health. High sodium consumption is a significant contributor to the development of hypertension (high blood pressure), which is a major risk factor for heart disease. Here's why managing sodium intake is important and how to do it effectively:

1. Sodium and Blood Pressure:

- Sodium is a mineral that is essential for various bodily functions, including maintaining fluid balance and supporting nerve and muscle function. However, excessive sodium intake can lead to higher blood pressure. This happens because sodium causes the body to retain water, which increases blood volume and, in turn, blood pressure.

2. Dietary Sources of Sodium:

- The primary source of dietary sodium comes from salt, or sodium chloride. High-sodium foods and sources include:
  - Processed and packaged foods (canned soups, frozen meals, snacks)
  - Restaurant and fast-food meals (often high in salt)
  - Bread and baked goods (some bread contains a significant amount of sodium)
  - Deli meats and processed meats (e.g., ham, bacon, sausages)
  - Condiments (soy sauce, salad dressings)
  - Salt added during cooking or at the table

3. Reducing Sodium Intake:

- To control blood pressure and reduce sodium intake, consider the following strategies:

  - **Read Food Labels:** Pay attention to the sodium amount on food labels. Choose "low-sodium" or "sodium-free" items whenever possible.

   - **Cook at Home:** You may regulate how much salt is added to your food when you prepare it at home. Experiment with herbs, spices, and other flavorings to reduce the reliance on salt for taste.

   - **Limit Processed Foods:** Reduce your intake of processed and packaged foods, which are generally rich in salt. Choose whole, fresh foods instead.

   - **Choose Low-Sodium Alternatives:** When shopping, select lower-sodium options for canned goods, soups, and other products.

   - **Avoid Excessive Salt at Restaurants:** When dining out, request that your meal be prepared with less salt. Take care when using sauces and condiments high in salt.

   - **Use Salt Sparingly:** When adding salt to your food, do so sparingly. Consider using less salt or using alternatives like potassium chloride (a salt substitute) if recommended by a healthcare professional.

   - **Rinse Canned Vegetables:** If you use canned vegetables, rinsing them under running water can help reduce their sodium content.

4. Hidden Sodium:

- Be aware of hidden sources of sodium in foods that may not taste salty, such as bread, cereal, and dairy products. Some of these products may contain significant amounts of sodium.

5. Gradual Reduction:

- Reducing sodium intake is often more effective when done gradually. Your taste buds can adapt to lower-sodium foods over time.

6. Be Salt Savvy:

- Pay attention to the terms used in food labels, such as "sodium-free," "very low sodium," and "reduced sodium." These labels can guide your choices.

7. Consider Potassium: Increasing dietary potassium, found in foods like fruits, vegetables, and legumes, can help counter the blood pressure-raising effects of sodium.

8. Regular Blood Pressure Monitoring:

- If you have concerns about blood pressure or hypertension, monitor your blood pressure regularly and consult with a healthcare professional. They can provide personalized guidance and recommend appropriate interventions for blood pressure control.

Controlling sodium intake is an important step in managing and preventing hypertension and reducing the risk of heart disease. It's part of a broader approach to heart-healthy living that includes a balanced diet, regular physical activity, and stress management.

FOODS THAT LOWER BLOOD PRESSURE

Certain foods can help lower blood pressure and support overall heart health. These foods are often part of a heart-healthy diet that emphasizes nutrients known to have a positive impact on blood pressure. Here are some foods that may help lower blood pressure:

1. **Leafy Greens:** Leafy greens such as spinach, kale, and Swiss chard are rich in potassium, which can help the body balance sodium levels and reduce blood pressure.

2. **Berries:** Blueberries, strawberries, and raspberries are high in antioxidants called flavonoids, which may contribute to blood pressure reduction.

3. **Beets:** Beets are a good source of nitrates, which can help dilate blood vessels and improve blood flow, potentially lowering blood pressure.

4. **Oats:** Oats are high in fiber, which can help reduce blood pressure. They also contain beta-glucans, which have been associated with improved heart health.

5. **Fatty Fish:** Fatty fish like salmon, mackerel, and sardines are rich in omega-3 fatty acids, which have been linked to lower blood pressure and improved heart health.

6. **Garlic:** Garlic contains allicin, a compound that may have blood pressure-lowering effects. It can be used in various dishes and as a seasoning.

7. **Bananas:** Bananas are a good source of potassium, which can help regulate blood pressure.

8. **Nuts and Seeds:** Almonds, walnuts, and flaxseeds are high in potassium, magnesium, and healthy fats, all of which can support lower blood pressure.

9. **Beans and Legumes:** Beans, lentils, and chickpeas are excellent sources of fiber and are low in sodium, making them heart-healthy choices.

10. **Low-Fat Dairy:** Low-fat or fat-free dairy products like yogurt are good sources of calcium and protein, which may contribute to blood pressure control.

11. **Pomegranates:** Pomegranate juice and seeds contain antioxidants called polyphenols, which have been associated with reduced blood pressure.

12. **Quinoa:** Quinoa is a whole grain rich in fiber and protein. It can be a healthy alternative to refined grains in your diet.

13. **Dark Chocolate:** Dark chocolate with a high cocoa content (70% or more) contains flavonoids that may help relax blood vessels and lower blood pressure. Consume it in moderation.

14. **Hibiscus Tea:** Some studies suggest that hibiscus tea may have blood pressure-lowering effects due to its natural compounds.

15. **Turmeric:** The active compound in turmeric, curcumin, may help lower blood pressure and reduce inflammation.

16. **Olive Oil:** Extra virgin olive oil is a source of monounsaturated fats, which can contribute to better heart health and potentially lower blood pressure.

It's important to note that individual responses to these foods may vary, and the effectiveness of dietary changes can depend on factors such as overall diet, genetics, and lifestyle. A balanced diet that includes a variety of these foods, along with a reduction in sodium intake, can be a key part of a comprehensive approach to blood pressure control. Always consult with a healthcare professional for personalized advice on managing your blood pressure and overall heart health.

CHAPTER SEVEN

MANAGING WEIGHT FOR HEART HEALTH

Managing weight is a crucial aspect of heart health, as excess body weight, especially when it leads to obesity, can significantly increase the risk of heart disease. Here are strategies for managing weight to support heart health:

1. **Balanced Diet:**
   - Adopt a balanced and heart-healthy diet that includes a variety of fruits, vegetables, whole grains, lean proteins, and healthy fats.
   - Reduce or eliminate high-calorie, low-nutrient foods and sugary beverages from your diet.
   - Practice portion control to avoid overeating and manage calorie intake.

2. **Regular Physical Activity:**
   - Engage in regular physical activity, including both aerobic exercises (e.g., walking, swimming, cycling) and strength training.
   - As advised by health guidelines, try to get at least 150 minutes a week of moderate-intensity aerobic exercise or 75 minutes of vigorous-intensity exercise.

- Strength training can help build muscle, which can boost metabolism and support weight management.

3. **Lifestyle Modifications:**
   - Get enough sleep, as sleep quality and duration can affect appetite and weight.
   - Manage stress through relaxation techniques like deep breathing, meditation, or yoga to prevent stress-related eating.
   - By identifying and regulating triggers, you can avoid mindless snacking and emotional eating.

4. **Hydration:**
   - Throughout the day, sip a lot of water. There are instances when people confuse thirst for hunger, which results in overindulging in calories.

5. **Set Realistic Goals:**
   - Establish achievable weight loss goals. Small, sustainable changes are more effective than extreme diets or rapid weight loss attempts.

6. **Consult a Healthcare Professional:**
   - If you have significant weight loss goals or underlying health conditions, consult with a healthcare professional or a registered dietitian for personalized guidance.

7. **Track Your Progress:**
   - Keep a food diary or use a mobile app to track your food intake and physical activity. This might

assist you in determining where you need to improve.

8. **Social Support:**
   - Share your goals with friends or family members and consider joining a weight loss or healthy lifestyle support group. Social support can be motivating and help you stay on track.

9. **Behavioral Strategies:**
   - Practice mindful eating, which involves paying full attention to your meals and savoring each bite. This can help prevent overeating.
   - Steer clear of distractions like TV and internet use during eating.

10. **Avoid Extreme Diets:**
   - Steer clear of fad diets and extreme weight loss methods, as they can be unsustainable and potentially harmful.

11. **Weight Maintenance:**
   - Once you achieve your desired weight, focus on weight maintenance by continuing to follow a balanced diet and exercise routine.

12. **Regular Check-Ups:**
   - Visit your healthcare provider for regular check-ups and screenings to monitor your heart health and overall well-being.

Remember that losing even a small amount of weight can lead to significant improvements in heart health. Every effort to maintain a healthy weight contributes to a reduced risk of heart disease, and it's a valuable investment in your overall well-being. Always seek guidance from healthcare professionals or registered dietitians when embarking on weight management efforts, as they can provide personalized recommendations tailored to your specific needs and goals.

THE CONNECTION BETWEEN WEIGHT AND HEART DISEASE

The connection between weight and heart disease is significant and well-established. Excess body weight, particularly when it leads to obesity, is a major risk factor for the development of various heart-related conditions. Here's an overview of the relationship between weight and heart disease:

1. **Obesity and Heart Disease:**
   - Having an excessive quantity of bodily fat is the definition of obesity. It is closely associated with an increased risk of heart disease, including coronary artery disease (CAD), heart attacks, heart failure, and arrhythmias (irregular heart rhythms).
   - Excess body fat, especially when concentrated around the abdomen (visceral fat), can lead to inflammation, insulin resistance, and dyslipidemia

(abnormal blood lipid levels), all of which contribute to heart disease risk.

2. **Hypertension (High Blood Pressure):**
   - Obesity is a significant contributor to high blood pressure, which is a major risk factor for heart disease. Excess body weight requires the heart to pump more blood, which can lead to increased pressure on the arterial walls.

3. **Dyslipidemia (Abnormal Blood Lipids):**
   - Obesity often leads to unfavorable changes in blood lipid profiles, including elevated levels of LDL cholesterol (the "bad" cholesterol) and triglycerides. It can also decrease HDL cholesterol (the "good" cholesterol).
   - These lipid abnormalities are associated with atherosclerosis (plaque buildup in arteries) and an increased risk of heart disease.

4. **Diabetes and Insulin Resistance:**
   - Obesity is a primary risk factor for the development of type 2 diabetes, a condition associated with insulin resistance. Diabetes significantly raises the risk of heart disease, as it can cause damage to blood vessels and increase the likelihood of heart attacks and strokes.

5. **Sleep Apnea:**
   - Obesity is a common cause of obstructive sleep apnea, a condition where breathing stops and starts during sleep. Sleep apnea is linked to

hypertension and increases the risk of heart
disease.

6. **Inflammation and Oxidative Stress:**
   - Excess body fat, particularly visceral fat,
promotes inflammation and oxidative stress in the
body. Chronic inflammation is a key factor in the
development of atherosclerosis and heart disease.

7. **Heart Failure:**
   - Obesity increases the risk of heart failure, a
condition where the heart's ability to pump blood is
compromised. The heart has to work harder to
support the extra weight, which can lead to heart
muscle damage over time.

8. **Atrial Fibrillation (AFib):**
   - Obesity is associated with a higher risk of
developing atrial fibrillation, an irregular heart
rhythm that can lead to stroke and heart failure.

9. **Stroke:**
   - Obesity is a risk factor for stroke, which is often
a result of vascular damage and blood clot
formation associated with excess weight.

10. **Treatment Challenges:**
   - Obesity can make the management of heart
disease more complex, as it may affect the
effectiveness of medications and the outcomes of
surgical interventions.

Given the strong link between obesity and heart disease, maintaining a healthy body weight through a balanced diet and regular physical activity is crucial for heart health. Weight management efforts, even modest weight loss, can have a significant impact on reducing the risk of heart disease and its associated complications. It's important to consult with healthcare professionals or registered dietitians for guidance and support when embarking on a weight management journey to improve heart health.

PRACTICAL TIPS FOR WEIGHT CONTROL

Practical tips for weight control involve making sustainable lifestyle changes that can help you achieve and maintain a healthy weight. Here are some practical strategies to help you manage your weight effectively:

1. **Set Realistic Goals:** Start with achievable goals. Aim to lose 1-2 pounds per week, which is a safe and sustainable rate of weight loss.

2. **Balanced Diet:** Adopt a balanced and varied diet that includes a mix of fruits, vegetables, whole grains, lean proteins, and healthy fats. This ensures you get essential nutrients while managing calorie intake.

3. **Portion Control:** Be mindful of portion sizes. To help control servings, use smaller plates and utensils. Avoid going back for seconds.

4. **Track Your Intake:** Keep a food diary or use mobile apps to record what you eat. This can assist you in becoming more conscious of your eating patterns.

5. **Eat Regular Meals:** Have regular, balanced meals and avoid skipping meals. Later in the day, this helps avoid overindulging.

6. **Mindful Eating:** Pay attention to your meals. Avoid eating in front of the TV or computer, and savor each bite. Eating thoughtfully can assist you in recognizing when you are full.

7. **Stay Hydrated:** Throughout the day, sip a lot of water. Sometimes, thirst is mistaken for hunger, leading to overindulgence in calories.

8. **Limit Sugary and Processed Foods:** Reduce your consumption of foods and beverages high in added sugars. Minimize processed and fast foods, as they are often high in calories and low in nutrients.

9. **Include Protein:** Incorporate protein-rich foods like lean meats, poultry, fish, beans, and dairy products into your meals. Protein might help you feel satiated and full.

10. **Fiber-Rich Foods:** Choose foods high in fiber, such as whole grains, fruits, and vegetables. Fiber can promote satiety and support healthy digestion.

11. **Meal Prep:** Plan and prepare meals in advance to have healthier options readily available. This might assist you in making healthier food choices.

12. **Healthy Snacking:** If you snack, choose healthy options like fruits, vegetables, yogurt, or nuts. Avoid mindless snacking.

13. **Limit Liquid Calories:** Be mindful of the calories in beverages. Choose water, herbal tea, or other low-calorie drinks over sugary drinks and excessive amounts of alcohol.

14. **Physical Activity:** Engage in regular physical activity. Make sure your schedule consists of both strength and cardio training exercises. Aim for 150 minutes or more of moderate-to-intense aerobic activity per week.

15. **Break Up Sedentary Time:** If you have a desk job or sit for extended periods, take breaks to stand, stretch, or walk.

16. **Find an Activity You Enjoy:** Choose physical activities that you enjoy, whether it's dancing,

hiking, or playing sports. This increases the likelihood that you will stay to your fitness plan.

17. **Social Support:** Share your goals with friends or family members. Think about joining a support group for healthy living or weight loss. Social support can be motivating.

18. **Sleep and Stress Management:** Prioritize good-quality sleep, as it can affect appetite and weight. Use relaxation methods to control your stress, such as yoga, meditation, or deep breathing.

19. **Regular Monitoring:** Track your progress, including your weight, body measurements, and fitness level. This can help you stay accountable and motivated.

20. **Consult a Healthcare Professional:** If you have specific weight management goals, consider consulting with a healthcare professional or a registered dietitian for personalized guidance and support.

Remember that healthy weight control is about making long-term, sustainable changes to your lifestyle. It's not just about losing weight but also maintaining a weight that promotes good health. Focus on gradual progress, and don't be too hard on yourself if you encounter setbacks. All of it is a necessary step on the path to improved health and wellbeing.

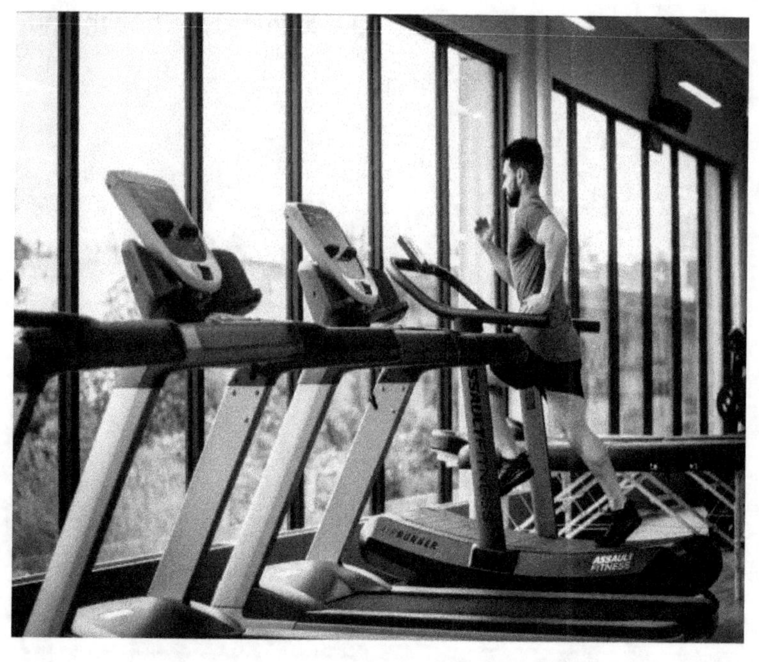

CHAPTER EIGHT

DIET AND DIABETES

Diet plays a crucial role in managing diabetes. Whether you have type 1 diabetes, type 2 diabetes, or are at risk of developing diabetes, making smart dietary choices can help regulate blood sugar levels and support your overall health. Here are some key points about diet and diabetes:

1. Carbohydrate Management:
  - The biggest influence on blood sugar levels is provided by carbohydrates. It's critical to control and observe how much carbohydrates you consume.
  - Focus on complex carbohydrates like whole grains, legumes, vegetables, and fruits, which provide steady energy and are rich in fiber.

2. Glycemic Index:
  - Pay attention to the glycemic index (GI) of foods. Low-GI foods cause a slower rise in blood sugar, while high-GI foods can cause rapid spikes.
  - Choose lower-GI foods like whole grains, non-starchy vegetables, and legumes.

3. Portion Control:
  - Use portion control to control how many calories and carbohydrates you eat.

   - Use measuring cups and a food scale to help
with portion accuracy.

4. Balanced Meals:
   - Strive for well-balanced meals that have a
healthy fat, carbohydrate, and lean protein source.
   - This can help stabilize blood sugar and provide
sustained energy.

5. Healthy Fats:
   - Make sure your diet contains healthy fats from
foods like avocados, nuts, seeds, and olive oil.
   - These fats can help control blood sugar and
improve heart health.

6. Sugar and Sweeteners:
   - Limit added sugars and sugary beverages, as
they can cause rapid blood sugar spikes.
   - Use sugar substitutes in moderation, if needed,
and consult with a healthcare professional.

7. Fiber-Rich Foods:
   - Consume plenty of fiber from fruits, vegetables,
whole grains, and legumes.
   - Fiber can enhance digestion and help control
blood sugar levels.

8. Regular Meals:
   - Eat regular, balanced meals and avoid skipping
meals. This helps prevent blood sugar fluctuations.

9. Snacking:

- Choose healthy snacks like yogurt, nuts, or vegetables with hummus to manage hunger and maintain blood sugar control.

10. Alcohol:
   - Drink alcohol sparingly and in conjunction with meals. Alcohol can cause blood sugar levels to fluctuate.

11. Consistency:
   - Consistency in your meal timing and carbohydrate intake can help stabilize blood sugar levels.

12. Monitoring and Testing:
   - Check your blood sugar levels on a regular basis as directed by your physician. Testing can help you understand how different foods and meals affect your blood sugar.

13. Individualized Plans:
   - Work with a registered dietitian or a diabetes educator to create a personalized meal plan that meets your specific needs and preferences.

14. Medications and Insulin:
   - If prescribed medications or insulin, take them as directed by your healthcare provider to manage blood sugar effectively.

15. Weight Management:

- If you have type 2 diabetes and are overweight, weight management through diet and physical activity is often a key part of treatment.

16. Consultation with a Healthcare Professional:
   - Always consult with a healthcare professional or registered dietitian for personalized guidance and adjustments to your diet plan.

Managing diabetes through diet is a lifelong journey that requires continuous monitoring and adaptation. The goal is to maintain stable blood sugar levels, prevent complications, and improve overall well-being. By making informed dietary choices and working closely with healthcare professionals, you can effectively manage diabetes and lead a healthy and fulfilling life.

DIABETES AS A HEART DISEASE RISK FACTOR

Heart disease is a substantial risk factor in diabetes. Individuals with diabetes, whether type 1 or type 2, are at an increased risk of developing cardiovascular conditions. Here's how diabetes contributes to heart disease risk:

1. **Atherosclerosis:** Diabetes can lead to the development of atherosclerosis, a condition where plaque builds up in the arteries. This plaque consists of cholesterol and other substances that

can narrow and block blood vessels. As a result, it becomes more difficult for blood to flow, which can lead to heart disease.

2. **High Blood Pressure:** People with diabetes are more likely to develop hypertension (high blood pressure), which is a major risk factor for heart disease. Elevated blood pressure puts additional stress on the heart and blood vessels.

3. **Abnormal Blood Lipids:** Diabetes often leads to unfavorable changes in blood lipid profiles, including elevated levels of LDL cholesterol (the "bad" cholesterol) and triglycerides. It can also decrease HDL cholesterol (the "good" cholesterol). These lipid abnormalities contribute to atherosclerosis.

4. **Insulin Resistance:** In type 2 diabetes, the body becomes resistant to the effects of insulin, leading to elevated blood sugar levels. A higher risk of heart disease is linked to insulin resistance.

5. **Inflammation:** Diabetes is linked to chronic inflammation in the body, which can damage blood vessels and contribute to the development of atherosclerosis.

6. **Microvascular Complications:** Diabetes can cause microvascular complications, such as damage to the small blood vessels in the heart.

This can lead to conditions like microvascular angina, which can cause chest pain and discomfort.

7. **Obesity:** While not all individuals with diabetes are overweight, there is a strong connection between obesity and type 2 diabetes. Obesity is an independent risk factor for heart disease.

8. **Hyperglycemia:** High blood sugar levels can damage blood vessels and lead to the formation of advanced glycation end products (AGEs), which can further contribute to atherosclerosis.

9. **Increased Risk of Heart Attacks:** Individuals with diabetes have a higher risk of heart attacks (myocardial infarctions) due to the combination of atherosclerosis and increased vulnerability of the heart muscle to ischemia (inadequate blood supply).

10. **Stroke:** Diabetes is a risk factor for stroke, which is another cardiovascular event closely related to heart disease.

Managing diabetes through lifestyle changes, medication, and blood sugar control is essential for reducing the risk of heart disease. Individuals with diabetes should work closely with healthcare professionals to monitor and manage their condition, including blood sugar levels, blood pressure, and blood lipid profiles. Lifestyle modifications, such as a heart-healthy diet, regular physical activity, and stress management, play a crucial role in reducing the impact of diabetes on heart health. It's important for individuals with diabetes to be proactive in managing both conditions to lower their risk of heart disease and its complications.

MANAGING BLOOD SUGAR THROUGH DIETS

Managing blood sugar through diet is a critical aspect of diabetes care. Whether you have type 1 diabetes, type 2 diabetes, or are at risk of developing diabetes, making the right dietary choices can help regulate blood sugar levels and improve overall health. Here are some key strategies for managing blood sugar through diet:

1. **Carbohydrate Management:**
   - The biggest influence on blood sugar levels is provided by carbohydrates. Pay close attention to the quantity and quality of carbohydrates in your diet.
   - Choose complex carbohydrates like whole grains, legumes, and vegetables, which have a lower impact on blood sugar. Limit simple carbohydrates like sugary foods and beverages.

2. **Glycemic Index (GI):**

- Understand the glycemic index of foods. Lower-GI foods cause a slower and more stable rise in blood sugar levels.
   - Favor low-GI foods, such as whole grains, non-starchy vegetables, and legumes.

3. **Portion Control:**
   - Pay attention to portion sizes to prevent consuming too many calories and carbs.
   - Use measuring cups and a food scale for accurate portion control.

4. **Balanced Meals:**
   - Aim for balanced meals that include lean protein sources, healthy fats, and carbohydrates. This helps prevent rapid blood sugar fluctuations.

5. **Regular Meal Timing:**
   - Have meals and snacks at regular intervals throughout the day. Spacing meals evenly can help regulate blood sugar levels.

6. **Fiber-Rich Foods:**
   - Increase the amount of high-fiber items in your diet, such as whole grains, legumes, fruits, and vegetables. Fiber can help stabilize blood sugar and improve digestion.

7. **Protein-Rich Foods:**
   - Include lean protein sources like poultry, fish, tofu, and beans in your meals. Protein can help maintain satiety and regulate blood sugar.

8. **Healthy Fats:**
   - Incorporate wholesome fats from foods like olive oil, avocados, almonds, and seeds. These fats can help control blood sugar and improve heart health.

9. **Limit Sugary Foods and Beverages:**
   - Minimize or avoid added sugars and sugary beverages, as they can lead to rapid blood sugar spikes.

10. **Snacking:**
   - Choose healthy snacks like yogurt, nuts, or vegetables with hummus to manage hunger and maintain blood sugar control.

11. **Hydration:**
   - To stay hydrated during the day, sip water. Sometimes, dehydration can affect blood sugar levels.

12. **Alcohol Moderation:**
   - If you consume alcohol, do so in moderation and with food, as it can impact blood sugar.

13. **Regular Monitoring:**
   - Keep an eye on your blood sugar levels as directed by your physician. This helps you understand how different foods affect your blood sugar.

14. **Individualized Meal Plan:**

- Work with a registered dietitian or a diabetes educator to create a personalized meal plan tailored to your specific needs and preferences.

15. **Carbohydrate Counting:**
   - Learn to count carbohydrates to accurately dose insulin (if applicable) and make informed food choices.

16. **Adjustments with Medications:**
   - If you're taking diabetes medications, follow your healthcare provider's instructions for medication use and dosage adjustments based on meals.

17. **Consultation with Healthcare Professionals:**
   - Always consult with your healthcare provider or a registered dietitian for personalized guidance and adjustments to your diet plan.

Managing blood sugar through diet is a lifelong commitment that requires continuous attention and adaptation. By making informed dietary choices and working closely with healthcare professionals, you can effectively regulate blood sugar levels and improve your overall well-being while living with diabetes.

THE ROLE OF CARBOHYDRATES

Carbohydrates play a crucial role in the human diet and have a significant impact on overall health, energy production, and blood sugar regulation. Here's an overview of the role of carbohydrates in the body:

1. **Primary Energy Source:**
   - The body uses carbohydrates as its main and most effective energy source. When consumed, carbohydrates are broken down into glucose, which is used by cells for fuel.
   - Glucose is particularly important for the brain, which relies on a continuous supply of glucose for its energy needs.

2. **Blood Sugar Regulation:**
   - Carbohydrates have a direct and significant impact on blood sugar (glucose) levels. Different carbohydrates have varying effects on blood sugar, depending on their glycemic index (GI).
   - Foods with a low GI cause a slow and steady increase in blood sugar, while those with a high GI lead to rapid spikes and crashes.

3. **Energy Storage:**
   - Excess glucose that is not immediately needed for energy is stored in the form of glycogen in the liver and muscles. When the body needs more energy, as it does during activity, glucose can be produced by breaking down glycogen.

4. **Muscle Function:**
   - Carbohydrates are essential for muscular contractions during physical activity. Athletes often

"carb-load" before endurance events to maximize glycogen stores.

5. **Brain Function:**
   - Glucose is the main energy source for the brain. A consistent supply of carbohydrates is necessary to support cognitive function.

6. **Digestive Health:**
   - Dietary fiber, a type of carbohydrate found in plant foods, is crucial for digestive health. It helps maintain regular bowel movements, prevents constipation, and supports a healthy gut microbiome.

7. **Micronutrient Sources:**
   - Many carbohydrate-rich foods, such as fruits, vegetables, and whole grains, are rich sources of essential vitamins and minerals. Consuming a variety of carbohydrates can help meet nutrient requirements.

8. **Fullness and Satiety:**
   - Carbohydrates can promote feelings of fullness and satiety. High-fiber carbohydrates can help control appetite and prevent overeating.

9. **Dietary Variety:**
   - Carbohydrates come in various forms, including sugars, starches, and fiber. They add variety and taste to the diet.

10. **Balanced Diet:**
   - A balanced diet includes carbohydrates along with proteins and fats to provide essential nutrients for overall health.

It is noteworthy that not every carbohydrate is made equal. While complex carbohydrates from whole foods like vegetables, fruits, legumes, and whole grains are generally considered healthy, simple carbohydrates from sugars and highly processed foods should be limited in the diet, especially for those concerned about blood sugar regulation.

For individuals with diabetes, understanding the types and amounts of carbohydrates in their diet is crucial for blood sugar management. Consultation with a healthcare provider or a registered dietitian can help individuals make informed dietary choices to achieve optimal blood sugar control while meeting their nutritional needs.

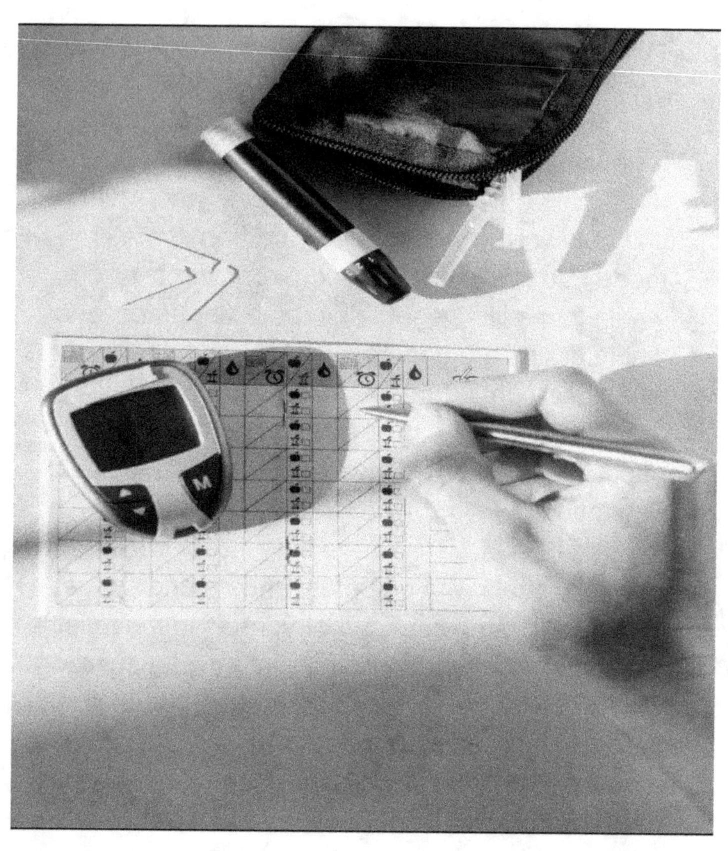

CHAPTER NINE

NUTRIENTS FOR HEART HEALTH

Maintaining heart health is vital for overall well-being, and a balanced diet can play a significant role in promoting cardiovascular health. Here are essential nutrients and dietary components that support heart health:

1. **Omega-3 Fatty Acids:**
   - Found in fatty fish (e.g., salmon, mackerel, sardines), flaxseeds, and walnuts, omega-3 fatty acids help reduce the risk of heart disease by lowering triglycerides, reducing inflammation, and supporting healthy blood vessels.

2. **Fiber:**
   - Dietary fiber, found in whole grains, fruits, vegetables, legumes, and nuts, can help lower cholesterol levels, regulate blood pressure, and improve digestion. Soluble fiber is particularly effective at reducing LDL cholesterol.

3. **Antioxidants:**
   - Antioxidants like vitamins C and E, as well as phytochemicals in fruits and vegetables, can protect the heart by reducing oxidative stress and

inflammation. Berries, citrus fruits, and green leafy
vegetables are rich sources.

4. **Potassium:**
   - By counteracting the effects of sodium on the
body, potassium helps control blood pressure. It's
abundant in foods like bananas, sweet potatoes,
and spinach.

5. **Magnesium:**
   - Magnesium is important for heart rhythm
regulation and blood pressure control. Leafy
greens, whole grains, nuts, and seeds are all good
sources.

6. **Calcium:**
   - Calcium plays a role in muscle contraction,
including the heart's muscle. It can be obtained
from dairy products, fortified plant-based milk, and
leafy greens.

7. **Folate (Vitamin B9):**
   - Folate supports heart health by reducing levels
of homocysteine, a compound linked to heart
disease. It's found in leafy greens, lentils, and
fortified cereals.

8. **Vitamin K:**
   - Vitamin K is important for blood clotting and
preventing the buildup of calcium in arteries.
Broccoli, Brussels sprouts, and leafy greens are
excellent sources.

9. **Vitamin D:**
   - Vitamin D is essential for calcium absorption
and has implications for heart health. Exposure to
sunlight, fatty fish, and fortified foods can provide
vitamin D.

10. **Selenium:**
   - Selenium is an antioxidant mineral that can
protect the heart. Nuts, whole grains, and lean
meats contain it.

11. **Phytosterols:**
   - Phytosterols, plant compounds found in foods
like nuts and whole grains, can help lower LDL
cholesterol levels.

12. **Monounsaturated and Polyunsaturated
Fats:**
   - These heart-healthy fats are found in olive oil,
avocados, nuts, and seeds. They can help lower
LDL cholesterol levels.

13. **Coenzyme Q10 (CoQ10):**
   - CoQ10 supports heart health by assisting in
energy production in cells. It can be found in small
amounts in organ meats and seafood or taken as a
supplement.

14. **Garlic:**

- Garlic contains allicin, a compound that can help lower blood pressure and reduce the risk of atherosclerosis.

15. **Flavonoids:**
   - Flavonoids, present in foods like dark chocolate, tea, and berries, have antioxidant and anti-inflammatory properties that support heart health.

16. **Low Sodium (Salt):**
   - Reducing sodium intake is important for managing blood pressure. Avoiding highly processed and salty foods is a key part of this strategy.

17. **Low Added Sugars:**
   - High sugar intake can contribute to obesity and insulin resistance, which are risk factors for heart disease. Reducing added sugars in the diet is beneficial.

18. **Low Trans Fats:**
   - Trans fats, often found in partially hydrogenated oils, should be minimized in the diet. They may increase the risk of heart disease and boost LDL cholesterol.

A heart-healthy diet should focus on whole, unprocessed foods, including plenty of fruits, vegetables, whole grains, lean proteins, and healthy fats. Reducing saturated fats, trans fats, sodium, and added sugars is crucial for heart health. It's essential to follow a balanced and varied diet to ensure that you receive all the nutrients your heart needs to function at its best. Always consult with a healthcare provider or registered dietitian for personalized guidance on maintaining heart health through diet.

ANTIOXIDANTS AND ANTI-INFLAMMATORY FOOD

Antioxidants and anti-inflammatory foods are essential components of a healthy diet that can help protect your cells and tissues from damage, reduce inflammation, and support overall well-being. Here's a list of some foods rich in antioxidants and known for their anti-inflammatory properties:

1. Berries:
   - Blueberries, strawberries, raspberries, and blackberries are packed with antioxidants like anthocyanins, which have anti-inflammatory effects.

2. Dark Leafy Greens:
   - Spinach, kale, and Swiss chard are excellent sources of vitamins, minerals, and antioxidants like lutein and zeaxanthin, which support eye health and have anti-inflammatory properties.

3. Fatty Fish:

  - Omega-3 fatty acids, which are abundant in
salmon, mackerel, and sardines, have strong
anti-inflammatory properties.

4. Nuts and Seeds:
  - Almonds, walnuts, flaxseeds, and chia seeds
provide healthy fats, fiber, and antioxidants that
reduce inflammation.

5. Turmeric:
  - Curcumin, the active compound in turmeric, is a
powerful anti-inflammatory and antioxidant agent. It
can be used in curries, soups, and teas.

6. Ginger:
  - Gingerol, an ingredient in ginger, has antioxidant
and anti-inflammatory qualities. It's often used in
cooking and as a remedy for various ailments.

7. Green Tea:
  - Green tea is rich in catechins, which are potent
antioxidants with anti-inflammatory effects.

8. Dark Chocolate:
  - Dark chocolate (with at least 70% cocoa
content) contains flavonoids, which can reduce
inflammation and protect the heart.

9. Tomatoes:
  - Tomatoes are high in lycopene, a powerful
antioxidant known for its anti-inflammatory

properties. Cooking tomatoes can increase lycopene absorption.

10. Olive Oil:
   - Extra virgin olive oil includes oleocanthal, an anti-inflammatory compound, and is high in monounsaturated fats.

11. Beets:
   - Beets are rich in betalains, which have antioxidant and anti-inflammatory properties.

12. Citrus Fruits:
   - Oranges, lemons, and grapefruits are high in vitamin C, a potent antioxidant that also supports the immune system.

13. Sweet Potatoes:
   - Sweet potatoes are loaded with beta-carotene, an antioxidant that converts to vitamin A in the body and has anti-inflammatory effects.

14. Onions and Garlic:
   - Onions and garlic contain allicin and quercetin, which have anti-inflammatory and antioxidant properties.

15. Avocados:
   - Avocados are a source of monounsaturated fats, vitamin E, and various antioxidants that support heart health and reduce inflammation.

16. Cherries:
   - Cherries, particularly tart cherries, are rich in anthocyanins and other antioxidants that have anti-inflammatory effects.

17. Peppers:
   - Bell peppers, especially red and yellow varieties, are high in vitamin C and antioxidants that reduce inflammation.

18. Broccoli:
   - Broccoli is a cruciferous vegetable rich in sulforaphane, an antioxidant with anti-inflammatory properties.

Incorporating these foods into your diet can help you maintain good health, reduce the risk of chronic diseases, and manage inflammation. A balanced diet that includes a variety of these antioxidant-rich and anti-inflammatory foods can have a positive impact on your overall well-being.

OMEGA-3 FATTY ACIDS

One essential form of polyunsaturated fat that is crucial to overall health is omega-3 fatty acids. Three forms of omega-3 fatty acids are distinguished:

1. **Alpha-linolenic acid (ALA):** ALA is a short-chain omega-3 fatty acid found in plant-based

sources like flaxseeds, chia seeds, and walnuts. The body can convert a small portion of ALA into longer-chain omega-3s, but the conversion is limited.

2. **Eicosapentaenoic acid (EPA):** EPA is a long-chain omega-3 fatty acid commonly found in fatty fish, such as salmon, mackerel, and sardines. EPA is well-known for its anti-inflammatory and cardiovascular effects.

3. **Docosahexaenoic acid (DHA):** DHA is another long-chain omega-3 fatty acid found in fatty fish. It is particularly important for brain health, eye health, and overall cognitive function.

Here are some key roles and benefits of omega-3 fatty acids:

1. Heart Health:
   - Omega-3 fatty acids, especially EPA and DHA, are associated with a reduced risk of heart disease. They can lower triglycerides, reduce inflammation, and improve blood vessel function.

2. Brain Health:
   - DHA in particular is necessary for cognitive function and brain growth. It plays a role in maintaining healthy brain structure and function throughout life.

3. Eye Health:

- DHA is a major component of the retina in the eye and is essential for maintaining good vision and preventing age-related macular degeneration.

4. Inflammation Reduction:
- Omega-3s have anti-inflammatory properties and can help reduce chronic inflammation, which is linked to many chronic diseases.

5. Joint Health:
- Omega-3 fatty acids may help reduce joint pain and improve symptoms in conditions like rheumatoid arthritis.

6. Mood and Mental Health:
- Some studies suggest that omega-3s, particularly EPA, may have a positive impact on mood disorders, such as depression and anxiety.

7. Pregnancy and Development:
- DHA is vital for fetal brain and eye development during pregnancy. It's also important for the development of a child's nervous system.

8. Skin Health:
- Omega-3s can help maintain healthy skin by reducing inflammation and supporting the skin's natural protective barrier.

9. Immune System Support:

- Omega-3s may help modulate the immune response and improve the body's ability to fight infections and diseases.

It's important to include omega-3 fatty acids in your diet through a variety of sources. Fatty fish, like salmon and mackerel, are excellent dietary sources of EPA and DHA. For those who don't consume fish, plant-based sources like flaxseeds, chia seeds, and walnuts can provide ALA. Omega-3 supplements, including fish oil and algae-based supplements, are also available for those who may not get enough through their diet.

Always consult with a healthcare professional before starting any new dietary supplements, especially if you have specific health concerns or conditions. A balanced diet that includes a variety of omega-3 sources can contribute to overall health and well-being.

FIBER AND ITS CARDIOVASCULAR BENEFITS

Dietary fiber is a carbohydrate that is not digested and is found in plant-based meals. It offers a wide range of health benefits, and its positive impact on cardiovascular health is well-documented. Here are the cardiovascular benefits of dietary fiber:

1. **Lowering Cholesterol Levels:**

- Soluble fiber, found in foods like oats, beans, and fruits, can help lower LDL (bad) cholesterol levels. It does so by binding to cholesterol particles and removing them from the body.

2. **Reducing Blood Pressure:**
   - High-fiber diets, particularly those rich in whole grains, legumes, and vegetables, have been associated with lower blood pressure. The effect may be due to the ability of fiber to improve blood vessel function and reduce inflammation.

3. **Improving Blood Sugar Control:**
   - Soluble fiber can assist to normalize blood sugar levels by slowing carbohydrate breakdown and absorption. This is especially advantageous for diabetics or those at risk of developing diabetes.

4. **Weight Management:**
   - Fiber-rich foods are often lower in calories and provide a feeling of fullness and satiety. Consuming fiber can help with weight management by reducing overall calorie intake.

5. **Reducing Inflammation:**
   - Chronic inflammation is a risk factor for heart disease. Some types of fiber have anti-inflammatory properties, which can help protect the cardiovascular system.

6. **Promoting Healthy Gut Microbiota:**

- Fiber feeds the good bacteria in the gut by acting as a prebiotic. A balanced gut microbiome is linked to better heart health.

7. **Reducing Risk of Stroke:**
   - High-fiber diets have been associated with a reduced risk of stroke, likely due to their positive effects on cholesterol levels, blood pressure, and inflammation.

8. **Preventing Atherosclerosis:**
   - Atherosclerosis is the term for plaque buildup in the arteries. A diet high in fiber can help prevent or slow the progression of atherosclerosis by reducing cholesterol and promoting heart-healthy blood vessel function.

To enjoy these cardiovascular benefits, it's important to incorporate a variety of fiber-rich foods into your daily diet. The following are some top-notch sources of dietary fiber:

- Whole grains (oats, whole wheat, barley, quinoa)
- Legumes (lentils, chickpeas, black beans)
- Fruits (apples, pears, berries)
- Vegetables (broccoli, carrots, Brussels sprouts)
- Nuts and seeds, such as flaxseeds, chia seeds, and almonds

Aim to consume at least 25-30 grams of dietary fiber per day, as recommended by dietary guidelines. Gradually increase your fiber intake to allow your digestive system to adapt and minimize digestive discomfort.

Remember that a well-rounded, balanced diet, along with regular physical activity and other heart-healthy lifestyle choices, can further support your cardiovascular health. Always consult with a healthcare provider or registered dietitian for personalized guidance on incorporating fiber-rich foods into your diet to promote heart health.

CHAPTER TEN

PRACTICAL DIETARY STRATEGIES

Practical dietary strategies are essential for maintaining a healthy and balanced diet. These strategies can help you make informed choices, improve your eating habits, and support your overall well-being. Here are some practical dietary strategies to consider:

1. **Portion Control:**
   - Be mindful of portion sizes. Reduce the size of your dishes, plates, and utensils to help you eat less and avoid overindulging.

2. **Meal Planning:**
   - Arrange your snacks and meals ahead of time. This can help you make healthier choices, reduce impulse eating, and save time and money.

3. **Balanced Meals:**
   - Try to incorporate different food categories into each meal. A balanced meal typically consists of lean protein, whole grains, plenty of vegetables, and a source of healthy fats.

4. **Smart Snacking:**

- Choose healthy snacks, such as yogurt, nuts, fruits, or vegetables with hummus, to satisfy your hunger between meals without resorting to unhealthy options.

5. **Hydration:**
   - Sip lots of water to stay hydrated during the day. Sometimes it's difficult to distinguish between thirst and hunger.

6. **Mindful Eating:**
   - Eat mindfully by savoring your food, eating slowly, and paying attention to hunger and fullness cues. During meals, stay away from distractions like TV and phones.

7. **Variety:**
   - Eat a diverse assortment of foods to guarantee that your diet contains a range of nutrients. Different foods offer different health benefits.

8. **Cook at Home:**
   - Cooking at home allows you to have control over the ingredients and preparation methods, making it easier to choose healthier options.

9. **Limit Processed Foods:**
   - Reduce your consumption of highly processed and fast foods, which are often high in added sugars, unhealthy fats, and sodium.

10. **Label Reading:**

- Learn to read food labels to understand the nutritional content and make informed choices when shopping for groceries.

11. **Meal Prep:**
   - Prepare and portion your meals in advance to have healthy options readily available, especially for busy days.

12. **Dine Out Mindfully:**
   - When eating at restaurants, choose healthier menu options, request dressings and sauces on the side, and avoid oversized portions.

13. **Moderation:**
   - In moderation, enjoy sweets and decadent dishes. It's okay to savor your favorite foods occasionally.

14. **Social Support:**
   - Share your dietary goals with friends and family, and seek their support In making healthier choices together.

15. **Stress Management:**
   - Learn effective stress coping skills, as this may lead to emotional eating. Techniques like meditation, yoga, and exercise can help.

16. **Physical Activity:**

- Exercise on a regular basis enhances a balanced diet. Make an effort to fit exercise into your everyday schedule.

17. **Record Keeping:**
   - Keep a food diary or use a smartphone app to track your meals and snacks. This can help you identify eating patterns and make improvements.

18. **Consultation with a Dietitian:**
   - If you have specific dietary goals or health concerns, consider consulting a registered dietitian for personalized guidance and support.

Remember that dietary changes are best made gradually to create sustainable habits. What works for one person may not work for another, so it's important to find a dietary approach that suits your individual needs and preferences. With these practical strategies, you can make positive changes to your diet and improve your overall health over time.

MEAL PLANNING FOR HEART HEALTH

Meal planning for heart health is an effective way to ensure that you're making heart-healthy food choices on a regular basis. Here's a step-by-step guide for creating a heart-healthy meal plan:

1. **Set Clear Goals:**
   - Determine your specific heart health goals, such as reducing cholesterol, managing blood pressure, or achieving a healthy weight. Your food planning will be guided by your goals.

2. **Consult a Healthcare Professional:**
   - If you have specific dietary needs or restrictions due to heart disease or other medical conditions, consult a healthcare provider or registered dietitian for personalized guidance.

3. **Assess Your Current Diet:**
   - Take a look at your current eating habits and identify areas where improvements can be made. Are you consuming too much saturated fat, sodium, or added sugars? Are you lacking in fruits and vegetables?

4. **Choose Heart-Healthy Foods:**
   - Focus on including foods that promote heart health, such as:
     - Fruits and vegetables: Aim for a variety of colors and types.
     - Whole grains: Opt for foods like whole wheat, brown rice, quinoa, and oats.
     - Lean proteins: Select sources like skinless poultry, fish, beans, and legumes.
     - Healthy fats: Use olive oil, nuts, seeds, and avocados in moderation.
     - Low-fat dairy or dairy alternatives: Choose options with reduced saturated fat.

- Fiber-rich foods: Include beans, lentils, and whole grains for added fiber.

5. **Portion Control:**
   - Pay attention to portion proportions to prevent overindulging. Use measuring cups and a food scale if necessary to ensure proper portions.

6. **Meal Structure:**
   - Create well-balanced meals with lots of veggies, nutritious grains, and lean protein. This can help regulate blood sugar levels and prevent overeating.

7. **Limit Sodium and Added Sugars:**
   - Minimize your consumption of high-sodium and sugary foods and drinks. Use herbs and spices for flavor instead of salt, and choose unsweetened beverages.

8. **Meal Diversity:**
   - Include a variety of foods in your meal plan to ensure you get a wide range of nutrients and antioxidants.

9. **Meal Timing:**
   - Aim to eat regular, evenly spaced meals and snacks to maintain stable blood sugar levels.

10. **Hydration:**
    - Sip plenty of water throughout the day to stay hydrated. Limit sugary and high-caffeine beverages.

11. **Meal Prep:**
   - Plan your meals and snacks in advance, and prepare healthy options that are easy to grab when you're busy.

12. **Read Labels:**
   - Pay attention to food labels to identify the amount of saturated fat, trans fat, and sodium in packaged foods.

13. **Dine Out Mindfully:**
   - When eating at restaurants, choose dishes that align with your heart-healthy goals. Request modifications to reduce unhealthy ingredients.

14. **Track Your Progress:**
   - Keep a food diary or use a smartphone app to monitor your food intake and assess your progress.

15. **Stay Informed:**
   - Stay up-to-date with the latest nutritional guidelines and research related to heart health.

16. **Consult a Dietitian:**
   - A trained dietician can offer individualized advice and meal programs made to fit your unique requirements and tastes.

Creating a heart-healthy meal plan doesn't mean sacrificing flavor or enjoyment. There are plenty of delicious and satisfying heart-healthy recipes and options to choose from. Remember to make gradual changes and celebrate your successes along the way to a healthier heart.

READING FOOD LABELS

Reading food labels is an important skill for making informed and healthy food choices. Food labels provide essential information about the nutritional content of a product, including serving size, calories, and the amounts of various nutrients. Here's how to read food labels effectively:

1. **Start with the Serving Size:**
   - The serving size tells you the amount of food the nutrition information is based on. Make sure to check how much you actually eat vs the serving size listed on the label.

2. **Calories:**
   - The amount of energy in a food is indicated by the number of calories per serving. Be mindful of your daily calorie intake and how many servings you consume.

3. **Check the Nutrients:**
   - Pay attention to the amounts of key nutrients, including:
     - **Total Fat:** Look at the total fat content and the breakdown into saturated and trans fats. Choose foods lower in saturated and trans fats.

- **Cholesterol:** Limit foods high in cholesterol, especially if you have heart health concerns.
- **Sodium:** Be aware of the sodium content, as excessive sodium can contribute to high blood pressure. Look for lower-sodium options.
- **Total Carbohydrates:** Consider the total carbohydrates and the breakdown into dietary fiber and sugars. Aim for foods with higher fiber and lower added sugars.
- **Protein:** Protein content can vary, and it's important to choose sources of lean protein.
- **Vitamins and Minerals:** Labels often list the percentages of daily values (DV) for various vitamins and minerals. These percentages are based on a 2,000-calorie diet and can help you assess the nutrient content.

4. **% Daily Value (DV):**
   - The % DV indicates how much a nutrient in a serving of food contributes to your daily intake based on a 2,000-calorie diet. It can help you determine whether a food is high or low in a particular nutrient.
   - A general guideline is to aim for foods with a DV of 5% or less for nutrients like saturated fat, sodium, and added sugars and 20% or more for nutrients like fiber, vitamins, and minerals.

5. **Ingredient List:**
   - To find out what's in the product, look through the ingredients list. The primary component is listed first and the other ingredients are listed in

descending order based on weight. Look out for added sugars, artificial additives, and preservatives.

6. **Allergen Information:**
   - Food labels often highlight common allergens like wheat, nuts, soy, dairy, and eggs. If you have allergies, this section is crucial for your safety.

7. **Health Claims:**
   - Be cautious of health claims on the packaging, as they can be marketing tactics. For accurate information, rely on the Nutrition Facts panel.

8. **Comparing Products:**
   - When shopping, compare the nutrition labels of different products to choose the healthier option. Pay attention to differences in serving sizes.

9. **Understanding Footnotes:**
   - The footnote at the bottom of the Nutrition Facts panel explains the recommended daily values for various nutrients based on a 2,000-calorie diet. Remember that your specific needs may vary.

10. **Consider Special Dietary Needs:**
    - If you have specific dietary requirements or health conditions, consult a healthcare provider or registered dietitian to interpret food labels in the context of your individual needs.

Reading food labels can help you make informed choices that align with your health and nutritional goals. It's a valuable skill for maintaining a balanced and healthy diet.

EATING OUT SMARTLY

Eating out can be enjoyable and convenient, but it can also present challenges when trying to make healthy choices. Here are some tips for eating out smartly while still enjoying delicious meals:

1. **Plan Ahead:**
   - Before you go, view the restaurant's online menu. Look for healthier options and plan your order in advance to avoid impulsive, less healthy choices.

2. **Choose the Right Restaurant:**
   - Select restaurants that offer a variety of menu items, including healthier choices. These days, a lot of eateries post nutritional data on their websites.

3. **Practice Portion Control:**
   - Restaurants often serve large portions. Consider sharing a dish with a dining companion, ordering an appetizer as your main course, or asking for a to-go box to pack up half your meal before you start eating.

4. **Start with a Salad or Soup:**

- A salad or broth-based soup as an appetizer can help control your appetite and reduce your total calorie intake.

5. **Opt for Lean Proteins:**
   - Choose dishes that feature lean protein sources like grilled chicken, fish, or legumes. Avoid fried or breaded options.

6. **Request Modifications:**
   - Don't be afraid to ask for substitutions or adjustments to your meal. For example, ask for dressing on the side, whole wheat bread instead of white, or steamed vegetables instead of fries.

7. **Mind Your Sides:**
   - Instead of high-calorie sides like french fries, choose healthier options like a side salad, fruit, or steamed vegetables.

8. **Watch the Sauces and Dressings:**
   - Dressings and sauces may include large amounts of bad fats and calories. To help you manage how much you use, ask to have them on the side.

9. **Be Mindful of Beverages:**
   - Water, unsweetened tea, or sparkling water are healthier choices than sugary sodas or high-calorie alcoholic beverages.

10. **Share Desserts:**

- If you want to enjoy dessert, share it with your dining companions to manage portion sizes.

11. **Limit Bread Baskets:**
   - If the restaurant serves bread or rolls before the meal, be cautious. It's easy to fill up on these before your main course arrives.

12. **Slow Down and Savor:**
   - Eat slowly, enjoy your meal, and pay attention to hunger and fullness cues. This can help prevent overeating.

13. **Skip the All-You-Can-Eat Buffets:**
   - Buffets can encourage overeating due to the abundance of food. If you do go, choose smaller portions and opt for healthier options.

14. **Be Wary of "Healthy" Labels:**
   - Some dishes labeled as "healthy" may still be high in calories or other less healthy ingredients. Review the full menu and nutrition information if available.

15. **Listen to Your Body:**
   - Pay attention to your body's signals of hunger and fullness. If you're satisfied after only one taste, don't feel obligated to finish it all.

16. **Special Dietary Needs:**
   - If you have specific dietary needs or food allergies, communicate them clearly with the

restaurant staff to ensure your meal meets your requirements.

17. **Enjoy Special Occasions:**
   - While it's important to make healthy choices when dining out, it's also okay to indulge on special occasions. Balance is key to a sustainable, enjoyable approach to eating out.

Remember that making smart choices when eating out is about balance and moderation. You can still enjoy restaurant meals while making choices that align with your health and nutrition goals.

CHAPTER ELEVEN

LIFESTYLE FACTORS AND HEART HEALTH

Heart health is significantly influenced by lifestyle variables. Making positive lifestyle choices can help reduce the risk of heart disease and improve overall cardiovascular well-being. Here are key lifestyle factors that impact heart health:

1. **Diet:**
   - A heart-healthy diet is crucial. Place a strong emphasis on entire grains, fruits, vegetables, lean meats, and healthy fats. Cut back on sodium, trans fats, added sweets, and saturated fats. A balanced diet supports weight management, blood pressure control, and healthy cholesterol levels.

2. **Physical Activity:**
   - Exercise on a regular basis is crucial for heart health. Aim for at least 150 minutes per week of moderate-intensity exercise or 75 minutes per week of strenuous exercise. Twice a week, incorporate strength training activities.

3. **Tobacco and Smoking:**
   - Smoking dramatically raises one's risk of heart disease. Quitting smoking can significantly improve

heart health. Avoid secondhand smoke exposure as well.

4. **Alcohol Consumption:**
   - Drinking too much alcohol can exacerbate cardiac issues. If you drink alcohol, do so in moderation (no more than one drink per day for women and two drinks for men).

5. **Weight Management:**
   - For heart health, it's critical to maintain a healthy weight. Losing excess weight can reduce the risk of heart disease and other related conditions, such as diabetes and high blood pressure.

6. **Stress Management:**
   - Persistent stress may be detrimental to the heart. Practice stress-reduction techniques like meditation, deep breathing, yoga, or hobbies to relax and unwind.

7. **Blood Pressure Control:**
   - Excessive blood pressure is one risk factor for heart disease. Monitor your blood pressure regularly and work with your healthcare provider to manage it through lifestyle changes and, if necessary, medication.

8. **Blood Sugar Control:**
   - High blood sugar levels (diabetes) can increase the risk of heart disease. Maintain blood sugar

within a healthy range through diet, exercise, and, if needed, medication.

9. **Sleep Quality:**
   - Strive for 7 to 9 hours of good sleep per night. Poor sleep can contribute to heart issues and increase the risk of cardiovascular disease.

10. **Regular Health Checkups:**
   - Visit your healthcare provider regularly for checkups and screenings to monitor heart health, cholesterol levels, and other risk factors.

11. **Social Connections:**
   - Strong social connections and support systems can positively impact heart health. Cultivate meaningful relationships and engage with friends and family.

12. **Sun Safety:**
   - Protect your skin from excessive sun exposure to prevent skin cancer, which can be linked to certain heart conditions.

13. **Environmental Exposures:**
   - Limit exposure to environmental toxins and pollutants, which can affect heart health.

14. **Medication Adherence:**
   - If you have been prescribed medications for heart health, take them as directed by your healthcare provider.

15. **Genetic Factors:**
   - Understand your family history of heart disease and discuss it with your healthcare provider for personalized risk assessment and prevention strategies.

Making positive lifestyle changes and adopting heart-healthy habits can significantly reduce the risk of heart disease and contribute to a longer, healthier life. Consult with a healthcare provider for personalized guidance and to create a plan tailored to your specific needs and risk factors.

THE ROLE OF PHYSICAL ACTIVITIES

Physical activity plays a crucial role in maintaining and improving heart health. Regular exercise offers a wide range of cardiovascular benefits, including:

1. **Strengthening the Heart Muscle:**
   - Exercise enhances the heart's capacity to pump blood. It can lead to a stronger and more efficient heart muscle, which means it can pump more blood with each beat.

2. **Lowering Blood Pressure:**
   - Regular physical activity can help reduce high blood pressure, which is a significant risk factor for heart disease.

3. **Improving Cholesterol Levels:**
   - Exercise can increase HDL (good) cholesterol and lower LDL (bad) cholesterol levels, contributing to better overall lipid profiles.

4. **Enhancing Blood Sugar Control:**
   - Exercise helps regulate blood sugar levels and can reduce the risk of developing type 2 diabetes, which is a risk factor for heart disease.

5. **Maintaining a Healthy Weight:**
   - Physical activity supports weight management by burning calories and building muscle. For the health of your heart, you must maintain a healthy weight.

6. **Reducing Inflammation:**
   - A persistent state of inflammation is linked to heart disease. Regular exercise can help reduce inflammation in the body.

7. **Enhancing Endothelial Function:**
   - Exercise can improve the function of the endothelium, the lining of blood vessels, promoting better blood flow and reducing the risk of atherosclerosis.

8. **Strengthening Lungs:**
   - Cardiovascular exercise strengthens the respiratory system, increasing lung capacity and improving oxygen delivery to the body.

9. **Promoting Vascular Health:**
   - Regular physical activity can help maintain
healthy blood vessels, preventing the development
of vascular diseases.

10. **Supporting Stress Reduction:**
   - Exercise is a natural stress reliever. Managing
stress is important for heart health, as chronic
stress can contribute to cardiovascular problems.

11. **Enhancing Overall Fitness:**
   - Improved cardiovascular fitness, as a result of
regular exercise, allows the heart to work more
efficiently during both rest and physical activity.

12. **Reducing the Risk of Blood Clots:**
   - Physical activity can help prevent the formation
of blood clots in arteries and veins, reducing the
risk of heart attacks and strokes.

13. **Lowering Triglycerides:**
   - Exercise can reduce triglyceride levels in the
blood, which is another factor linked to heart
disease.

14. **Boosting Mood and Mental Health:**
   - Regular physical activity can have a positive
impact on mental health, reducing the risk of
depression and anxiety, which can indirectly affect
heart health.

15. **Improving Sleep Quality:**

- Regular exercise can lead to better sleep, which is important for heart health.

To reap these benefits, aim for a combination of aerobic exercises (like brisk walking, running, cycling, or swimming) and strength training exercises (like weight lifting or bodyweight exercises). The American Heart Association suggests engaging in muscle-strengthening activities at least twice a week in addition to 150 minutes of moderate-intensity aerobic exercise or 75 minutes of vigorous-intensity aerobic activity per week.

It's important to choose activities you enjoy and can sustain over time. Always consult with a healthcare provider before starting a new exercise program, especially if you have underlying health conditions or concerns.

SMOKING CESSATION

Smoking cessation, or quitting smoking, is one of the most important steps you can take to improve your heart health and overall well-being. Smoking is a major risk factor for heart disease, and quitting can have immediate and long-term benefits for your cardiovascular health. Here are steps and strategies to help you quit smoking:

1. **Set a Quit Date:**

- Decide on a deadline to stop smoking.
 Having a target date can help you mentally
prepare for the change.

2. **Seek Support:**
   - Inform your loved ones of your decision to
resign and solicit their support. Consider joining a
support group or reaching out to a counselor or
healthcare provider for guidance.

3. **Identify Triggers:**
   - Recognize the situations, emotions, or habits
that trigger your smoking. This awareness can help
you develop strategies to cope with these triggers
without cigarettes.

4. **Consider Nicotine Replacement Therapy
(NRT):**
   - Nicotine replacement products, such as nicotine
gum, patches, or lozenges, can help reduce
withdrawal symptoms. Consult with a healthcare
provider to determine which NRT is right for you.

5. **Prescription Medications:**
   - Some prescription medications, like varenicline
(Chantix) or bupropion (Zyban), can help reduce
cravings and withdrawal symptoms. Talk with your
healthcare professional about these possibilities.

6. **Behavioral Therapy:**
   - Cognitive-behavioral therapy (CBT) and other
counseling techniques can be effective in helping

you change your smoking habits and cope with cravings.

7. **Plan for Stress Management:**
   - Develop healthy ways to manage stress, as stress can be a trigger for smoking. Exercise, meditation, deep breathing, and relaxation techniques can be helpful.

8. **Create a Smoke-Free Environment:**
   - Remove cigarettes, lighters, and ashtrays from your home, car, and workplace. Make your environment as smoke-free as possible.

9. **Stay Active:**
   - Engage in physical activities that can distract you from cravings and boost your mood.

10. **Use Apps and Online Resources:**
    - There are many smartphone apps and online resources designed to support smoking cessation. They can provide tips, tracking tools, and motivation.

11. **Celebrate Milestones:**
    - Celebrate your achievements along the way. Set small goals and reward yourself for each success.

12. **Stay Persistent:**
    - Don't be discouraged by setbacks. Many people need multiple attempts to quit smoking

before succeeding. Keep trying and take lessons from your experiences.

13. **Think About the Benefits:**
   - Remind yourself of the numerous health benefits of quitting, including improved heart health, increased life expectancy, and financial savings.

14. **Get Professional Help:**
   - If you're finding it extremely challenging to quit on your own, consider seeking the help of a healthcare provider or smoking cessation program.

Quitting smoking can be difficult, but the benefits for your heart and overall health are immense. Making the decision to give up is always a good idea, and it's never too late. Your heart and body will thank you for making this positive change.

STRESS MANAGEMENT

Effective stress management is vital for heart health and overall well-being. Chronic stress can contribute to heart disease and exacerbate other health conditions. Here are strategies to help you manage and reduce stress:

1. **Identify Stressors:**
   - Recognize the sources of your stress. Understanding what's causing stress is the first step in addressing it.

2. **Practice Relaxation Techniques:**
   - Techniques like deep breathing, meditation, progressive muscle relaxation, and guided imagery can help calm the mind and reduce stress.

3. **Regular Exercise:**
   - Exercising is an excellent method to unwind. Endorphins, which naturally elevate mood, are released by it. Try to get in at least 150 minutes a week of moderate-to-intense activity.

4. **Healthy Diet:**
   - A healthy diet can assist your body in managing stress. Avoid excessive caffeine, sugar, and alcohol, as they can exacerbate stress and anxiety.

5. **Adequate Sleep:**
   - Make an effort to obtain seven to nine hours of restful sleep each night. Sleep is crucial for emotional well-being and stress management.

6. **Time Management:**
   - Prioritize and arrange your everyday responsibilities. Effective time management can help reduce overwhelming feelings.

7. **Set Realistic Goals:**
   - Maintain a realistic perspective on your abilities. Setting unattainable goals can lead to stress.

8. **Social Support:**

- Continue to have a solid support system of friends and family. Emotional relief might come from talking to people about your thoughts and feelings.

9. **Engage in Relaxing Activities:**
   - Activities you enjoy, such as reading, gardening, painting, or listening to music, can be effective stress reducers.

10. **Limit Technology Use:**
   - Reduce screen time, particularly before bedtime, to prevent information overload and improve sleep quality.

11. **Practice Mindfulness and Mindful Eating:**
   - Be present in the moment, and savor your meals. Mindful eating can enhance your enjoyment of food and reduce stress.

12. **Seek Professional Help:**
   - If you find it difficult to manage stress on your own, consider speaking with a therapist or counselor. They can offer assistance and coping mechanisms.

13. **Positive Self-Talk:**
   - Replace negative self-talk with positive affirmations. This can increase resilience and self-worth.

14. **Hobbies and Interests:**

- Engage in hobbies and interests that bring you joy and a sense of accomplishment.

15. **Laugh More:**
   - Laughter is a natural stress reducer. Watch a funny movie, read a humor book, or spend time with people who make you laugh.

16. **Limit Exposure to Stressors:**
   - If certain situations or people consistently cause stress, consider limiting your exposure to them when possible.

17. **Journaling:**
   - Writing in a journal is a therapeutic technique to communicate your feelings and ideas.

18. **Learn to Say No:**
   - Avoid overcommitting yourself. It's okay to decline additional responsibilities or obligations.

19. **Practice Gratitude:**
   - Focus on what you're grateful for. This can calm you down and change your viewpoint.

20. **Progressive Muscle Relaxation:**
   - To relieve physical tension, this technique entails tensing and relaxing various muscle groups.

Remember that stress management is a personal journey, and what works best for one person may not be the same for another. Experiment with different strategies to find the combination that helps you manage stress effectively and protect your heart health.

CHAPTER TWELVE

DIAGNOSTIC TEST FOR HEART HEALTH

Diagnostic tests for heart health are crucial for assessing your cardiovascular well-being, identifying risk factors, and diagnosing heart conditions. These tests help healthcare professionals make informed decisions about your heart health and treatment options. Here are some common diagnostic tests:

1. **Blood Pressure Measurement:**
   - Regular blood pressure measurements help monitor your risk of hypertension, a significant risk factor for heart disease.

2. **Cholesterol Blood Test:**
   - A lipid panel measures cholesterol levels, including LDL (bad) cholesterol, HDL (good) cholesterol, and triglycerides. Elevated cholesterol levels can increase heart disease risk.

3. **Electrocardiogram (ECG or EKG):**
   - The electrical activity of the heart is measured in this examination. It's used to detect irregular heart rhythms (arrhythmias) and signs of previous heart attacks.

4. **Echocardiogram:**
   - An echocardiogram makes images of the heart using sound waves. It can help diagnose heart valve problems, heart muscle issues, and congenital heart defects.

5. **Stress Test:**
   - Stress tests evaluate how your heart responds to physical stress, usually through exercise or medication. They help diagnose coronary artery disease and assess heart function.

6. **Holter Monitor or Event Recorder:**
   - These portable devices record the heart's electrical activity over an extended period, helping diagnose intermittent arrhythmias.

7. **Cardiac Catheterization:**
   - This procedure involves threading a thin tube (catheter) through blood vessels to the heart. It's used to diagnose and treat coronary artery disease and other heart conditions.

8. **Coronary Angiography:**
   - A type of cardiac catheterization, it provides detailed images of the coronary arteries to evaluate blockages or narrowing.

9. **CT or MRI Angiography:**
   - These imaging tests can visualize the heart and blood vessels to detect heart disease, aneurysms, and other issues.

10. **Nuclear Stress Test:**
   - This test combines a stress test with the injection of a small amount of radioactive material to create images of blood flow to the heart.

11. **Blood Tests:**
   - Various blood tests can assess heart health, including markers of inflammation, cardiac enzymes (troponin), and brain natriuretic peptide (BNP) levels.

12. **Carotid Ultrasound:**
   - This test uses ultrasound to evaluate the carotid arteries in the neck for blockages that may increase stroke risk.

13. **Ankle-Brachial Index (ABI):**
   - ABI compares blood pressure in the arms and legs to detect peripheral artery disease (PAD).

14. **Calcium Scoring:**
   - This CT scan measures the amount of calcium in the coronary arteries, helping assess the risk of coronary artery disease.

15. **Electrophysiology Studies:**
   - These tests evaluate electrical activity in the heart and are used to diagnose and treat arrhythmias.

16. **Genetic Testing:**

- Genetic tests can identify genetic factors that may increase your risk of inherited heart conditions.

17. **Tilt Table Test:**
- This test assesses how your body responds to changes in position and can help diagnose conditions like vasovagal syncope.

The specific tests you may need depend on your risk factors, symptoms, and medical history. It's essential to consult with a healthcare provider to determine the most appropriate diagnostic tests for your heart health. Regular check-ups and early detection can play a critical role in preventing and managing heart conditions.

MEDICAL AND SURGICAL INTERVENTIONS

Medical and surgical interventions play a vital role in the treatment and management of various heart conditions and cardiovascular diseases. These interventions are prescribed based on the specific diagnosis and severity of the condition. Here are some common medical and surgical interventions for heart health:

Medical Interventions:

1. **Medications:**

- Medications are frequently prescribed to manage heart conditions. Common drugs include:
    - **Antiplatelet agents:** Such as aspirin to prevent blood clots.
    - **Beta-blockers:** to lower blood pressure and heart rate.
    - **Angiotensin-converting enzyme (ACE) inhibitors:** For managing high blood pressure and heart failure.
    - **Statins:** To lower cholesterol levels.
    - **Anticoagulants:** To prevent blood clot formation.
    - **Diuretics:** For managing fluid retention.
    - **Vasodilators:** To widen blood vessels and reduce blood pressure.
    - **Antiarrhythmic drugs:** To manage irregular heart rhythms.

2. **Cardiac Rehabilitation:**
   - This program combines exercise, education, and counseling to help individuals recover from heart-related events or procedures.

3. **Lifestyle Modifications:**
   - Changes in diet, exercise, smoking cessation, and stress management are essential components of managing heart health.

4. **Pacemaker:**
   - A pacemaker is an implanted device that helps regulate the heartbeat in cases of irregular heart rhythms (arrhythmias).

5. **Implantable Cardioverter-Defibrillator (ICD):**
   - An ICD is implanted in individuals at risk of life-threatening arrhythmias. It can shock people with electricity to get their hearts back to normal.

6. **Cardiac Medications:**
   - Medications like nitroglycerin can help manage chest pain (angina).

Surgical Interventions:

1. **Angioplasty and Stent Placement:**
   - Percutaneous coronary intervention (PCI) involves using a balloon to widen narrowed or blocked coronary arteries and placing a stent to keep the artery open.

2. **Coronary Artery Bypass Grafting (CABG):**
   - CABG is a surgical procedure to create new routes for blood flow when coronary arteries are severely blocked. This is frequently called "bypass surgery."

3. **Valve Replacement or Repair:**
   - Surgery can replace or repair heart valves that are not functioning correctly.

4. **Aneurysm Repair:**
   - Aneurysm surgery can repair weakened areas of blood vessels to prevent rupture.

5. **Heart Transplant:**
   - In cases of severe heart failure, a heart transplant may be necessary to replace a failing heart with a healthy donor heart.

6. **Ventricular Assist Device (VAD):**
   - A mechanical device called a VAD aids in the heart's blood pumping. It may be used as a bridge to transplant or as destination therapy for individuals who are not eligible for transplantation.

7. **Maze Procedure:**
   - This surgical intervention is used to treat atrial fibrillation (AFib) by creating a pattern of scar tissue in the heart to block abnormal electrical pathways.

8. **Myectomy:**
   - Myectomy is a surgical procedure used to treat hypertrophic cardiomyopathy by removing excess heart muscle that obstructs blood flow.

9. **Carotid Endarterectomy:**
   - This procedure removes plaque from the carotid arteries to reduce the risk of stroke.

10. **Heart Surgery for Congenital Heart Defects:**
   - Pediatric and adult congenital heart surgeries address structural heart issues present from birth.

The choice between medical and surgical interventions depends on the individual's condition, overall health, and specific needs. It is essential to work closely with a healthcare provider to determine the most appropriate intervention and create a tailored treatment plan. Advances in medical and surgical techniques continue to improve outcomes and quality of life for individuals with heart conditions.

MEDICATIONS AND THEIR ROLES

Medications are often prescribed to manage various heart conditions and cardiovascular risk factors. These medications play specific roles in improving heart health and addressing related issues. Here are common medications and their roles:

1. Antiplatelet Agents:
   - Examples: Aspirin, Clopidogrel, Prasugrel, Ticagrelor
   - Role: These drugs prevent the formation of blood clots by inhibiting platelet aggregation. They are commonly used to reduce the risk of heart attacks and strokes, especially in individuals with atherosclerosis or a history of such events.

2. Beta-Blockers:
   - Examples: Metoprolol, Atenolol, Carvedilol
   - Role: Beta-blockers reduce the heart's workload by slowing the heart rate and lowering blood pressure. They are often prescribed for

hypertension, heart failure, and to manage
arrhythmias.

**3. Angiotensin-Converting Enzyme (ACE)
Inhibitors:**
   - Examples: Lisinopril, Enalapril, Ramipril
   - Role: ACE inhibitors relax blood vessels and
reduce blood pressure. They are commonly used to
treat high blood pressure, heart failure, and certain
heart conditions.

4. Angiotensin II Receptor Blockers (ARBs):
   - Examples: Losartan, Valsartan, Irbesartan
   - Role: ARBs also relax blood vessels and lower
blood pressure. They are prescribed for similar
conditions as ACE inhibitors.

5. Statins:
   - Examples: Atorvastatin, Simvastatin,
Rosuvastatin
   - Role: Statins lower cholesterol levels in the
blood by inhibiting the production of LDL (bad)
cholesterol. They are used to reduce the risk of
atherosclerosis, heart attacks, and strokes.

6. Anticoagulants:
   - Examples: Warfarin, Dabigatran, Rivaroxaban,
Apixaban
   - Role: Anticoagulants reduce the risk of blood
clot formation and are used in conditions like atrial
fibrillation, deep vein thrombosis, and pulmonary
embolism.

7. Diuretics:
   - Examples: Hydrochlorothiazide, Furosemide
   - Role: Diuretics promote the removal of excess salt and water from the body, reducing fluid retention and lowering blood pressure. They treat hypertension and heart failure.

8. Calcium Channel Blockers:
   - Examples: Amlodipine, Verapamil, Diltiazem
   - Role: These drugs relax blood vessels and reduce the heart's workload. They are used to treat high blood pressure, angina, and certain arrhythmias.

9. Nitrates:
   - Examples: Nitroglycerin, Isosorbide dinitrate
   - Role: Nitrates relax and dilate blood vessels, improving blood flow. They are often used to relieve angina symptoms and manage heart conditions.

10. Antiarrhythmic Drugs:
   - Examples: Amiodarone, Flecainide, Sotalol
   - Role: Antiarrhythmic medications help regulate heart rhythm by preventing or managing irregular heartbeats (arrhythmias).

11. Vasodilators:
   - Examples: Hydralazine, Nitroprusside
   - Role: Vasodilators relax and expand blood vessels, reducing the workload on the heart. They

are used in heart failure and hypertensive emergencies.

12. Heart Failure Medications:
   - Examples: Digoxin, Sacubitril/valsartan, Spironolactone
   - Role: Medications specifically for heart failure may improve symptoms, reduce fluid retention, and enhance heart function.

13. Cholesterol Absorption Inhibitors:
   - Example: Ezetimibe
   - Role: These drugs reduce the absorption of dietary cholesterol from the digestive tract and are used to lower LDL cholesterol.

The specific medication and dosage depend on an individual's condition, risk factors, and overall health. It is essential to work closely with a healthcare provider to determine the most appropriate medication and treatment plan. Adhering to prescribed medications and regular follow-up with a healthcare provider are crucial for managing heart health effectively.

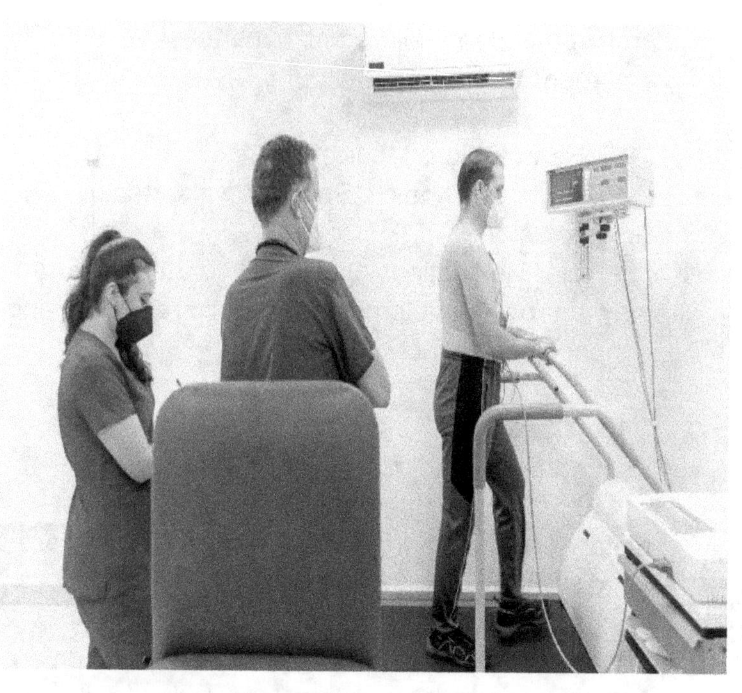

CHAPTER THIRTEEN

HEART HEALTHY BREAKFAST

A heart-healthy breakfast sets the tone for your day by providing essential nutrients and energy while supporting cardiovascular well-being. Here's a heart-healthy breakfast idea:

Oatmeal with Berries and Almonds:

Ingredients:
- 1/2 cup of rolled oats
- 1 cup of low-fat milk (or a dairy-free alternative like almond milk)
- Fresh berries (blueberries, strawberries, raspberries) 1/2 cup
- 1 tablespoon of sliced almonds
- 1 teaspoon (optional) honey or maple syrup

Instructions:
1. Place the milk and the rolled oats in a saucepan.
2. Cook over medium heat, stirring occasionally, until the oats have absorbed the milk and the mixture thickens (about 5-7 minutes).
3. After turning off the heat, scoop the oats into a bowl.
4. Top with fresh berries and sliced almonds.
5. Drizzle a small amount of honey or maple syrup over the oatmeal for added sweetness (optional).

This breakfast provides heart-healthy components:

- **Oats:** Because soluble fiber is abundant in oats, it may help reduce levels of LDL (bad) cholesterol.
- **Berries:** Berries are packed with antioxidants and fiber, which support heart health.
- **Almonds:** Almonds contain healthy fats and are a source of vitamin E, which is good for heart health.
- **Low-Fat Milk or Almond Milk:** These provide calcium and protein without the saturated fat found in whole milk.

Remember to adjust portion sizes and ingredients to meet your specific dietary needs and consult with a healthcare provider or registered dietitian for personalized dietary recommendations.

NUTRITIOUS LUNCHES AND DINNER

Nutritious lunches and dinners are essential for maintaining heart health. Here are some heart-healthy meal ideas for both lunch and dinner:

Lunch:

1. **Grilled Chicken Salad:**
   - Combine grilled chicken breast with a variety of colorful veggies (e.g., spinach, cherry tomatoes, cucumbers, bell peppers) and a light vinaigrette.

2. **Quinoa and Chickpea Salad:**
   - Toss cooked quinoa with chickpeas, diced cucumbers, cherry tomatoes, fresh herbs, and a lemon-tahini dressing.

3. **Mediterranean Wrap:**
   - Fill whole-grain wraps with lean protein (such as grilled chicken or tofu), hummus, fresh vegetables, and a sprinkle of feta cheese.

4. **Salmon and Brown Rice Bowl:**
   - Serve grilled or baked salmon on a bed of cooked brown rice with steamed broccoli and a drizzle of olive oil.

Dinner:

5. **Baked Salmon with Asparagus:**
   - Season salmon fillets with herbs and bake them alongside asparagus spears. Serve with a squeeze of lemon.

6. **Vegetable Stir-Fry:**
   - Stir-fry a mix of colorful vegetables (bell peppers, broccoli, carrots) with lean protein (chicken, tofu) and a low-sodium soy sauce. Serve over brown rice or quinoa.

7. **Tomato and Basil Whole Wheat Pasta:**

   - Toss whole wheat pasta with fresh tomatoes, basil, garlic, and a drizzle of olive oil. Top with a sprinkle of Parmesan cheese.

8. **Lentil and Vegetable Soup:**
   - Prepare a hearty soup with lentils, various vegetables, and low-sodium vegetable broth. Season with herbs and spices.

Remember these general tips for heart-healthy meals:

- Select lean proteins such as fish, lentils, and skinless chicken.
- Choose whole grains like quinoa, brown rice, and whole wheat pasta.
- Use healthy fats like olive oil and avocado instead of saturated or trans fats.
- Limit sodium intake by using herbs and spices for flavor.
- Include plenty of fruits and vegetables in your meals for fiber and antioxidants.
- Drink water and herbal teas to stay hydrated.

Tailor your meals to your specific dietary needs, and consult with a healthcare provider or a registered dietitian for personalized guidance on heart-healthy eating.

Snacks and desserts can also be part of a heart-healthy diet when chosen wisely. Here are some heart-healthy snack and dessert ideas:

Snacks:

1. **Mixed Nuts:**
   - A small handful of unsalted mixed nuts, such as almonds, walnuts, and pistachios, provides healthy fats and protein.

2. **Hummus and Veggies:**
   - Pair hummus with carrot and celery sticks, cherry tomatoes, and cucumber slices for a crunchy and nutritious snack.

3. **Greek Yogurt with Berries:**
   - Enjoy Greek yogurt topped with fresh berries like blueberries or raspberries for a protein-rich and antioxidant-packed snack.

4. **Apple Slices with Almond Butter:**
   - Slice apples and dip them in almond butter for a satisfying and heart-healthy combination.

5. **Air-Popped Popcorn:**
   - Make air-popped popcorn and season it with a sprinkle of herbs or nutritional yeast for flavor without excessive salt or butter.

Desserts:

6. **Dark Chocolate-Dipped Strawberries:**
   - Dip fresh strawberries in dark chocolate for a heart-healthy dessert with antioxidants.

7. **Baked Apples with Cinnamon:**
   - Core apples, sprinkle with cinnamon, and bake until tender. Top with a spoonful of Greek yogurt and serve.

8. **Chia Seed Pudding:**
   - Mix chia seeds with unsweetened almond milk, a touch of honey, and your favorite berries. Place it in the fridge for several hours or perhaps overnight.

9. **Frozen Yogurt with Fruit:**
   - Opt for low-fat frozen yogurt and top it with sliced peaches, strawberries, or other favorite fruits.

10. **Sorbet:**
   - Enjoy fruit sorbet, which is typically lower in fat than ice cream and comes in a variety of flavors.

Remember to moderate portion sizes and choose options that are lower in added sugars and unhealthy fats. Whenever feasible, use whole foods and natural sweeteners. Desserts can be a treat within a heart-healthy diet, so enjoy them in moderation.

CONCLUSION

In conclusion, maintaining heart health is a lifelong journey that requires a combination of healthy lifestyle choices, a nutritious diet, regular exercise, and ongoing medical management. Here are some key takeaways:

1. **Understanding Heart Health:** Heart health is crucial for overall well-being, and understanding the risk factors and common heart conditions is the first step in maintaining a healthy heart.

2. **Diet and Heart Health:** A heart-healthy diet is rich in fruits, vegetables, whole grains, lean proteins, and healthy fats. It's essential to limit saturated and trans fats, cholesterol, and sodium.

3. **Exercise:** Regular physical activity, including both aerobic and strength training, supports heart health by improving circulation and reducing the risk of heart disease.

4. **Weight Management:** Maintaining a healthy weight is vital for heart health, as excess weight can increase the risk of heart disease.

5. **Stress Management:** Effective stress management techniques can help reduce the impact of chronic stress on heart health.

6. **Medical and Surgical Interventions:**
Medications and surgical procedures are vital for
managing heart conditions and cardiovascular risk
factors. Adhering to prescribed treatments is
crucial.

7. **Regular Check-Ups:** Routine medical
check-ups and diagnostic tests are essential for
monitoring heart health, identifying risk factors, and
taking preventive measures.

8. **Lifestyle Choices:** Choices like quitting
smoking, limiting alcohol intake, and getting enough
quality sleep are integral to maintaining a healthy
heart.

9. **Dietary Strategies:** Incorporating
heart-healthy foods, managing cholesterol levels,
and controlling blood pressure through diet are key
components of heart health.

10. **Snacks and Desserts:** Snacks and desserts
can be part of a heart-healthy diet when chosen
wisely and in moderation.

Remember that heart health is a personal journey,
and it's essential to consult with healthcare
providers and registered dietitians for personalized
guidance and recommendations based on your
specific needs and risk factors. By making informed
choices and prioritizing your cardiovascular

well-being, you can enjoy a healthier and longer life with a strong and resilient heart.

EMPOWERING YOURSELF FOR HEART-HEALTHY LIVING

Empowering yourself for heart-healthy living is a proactive and essential approach to maintaining cardiovascular well-being. Here are some steps to help you take charge of your heart health:

1. **Education:** Knowledge is the foundation of empowerment. Educate yourself about heart health, risk factors, and common heart conditions. Understand the impact of lifestyle choices on your heart.

2. **Regular Check-Ups:** Schedule regular check-ups with your healthcare provider. These visits help monitor your heart health, identify risk factors, and make necessary adjustments to your treatment plan.

3. **Know Your Numbers:** Be aware of your key health numbers, including blood pressure, cholesterol levels, and blood sugar. Tracking these numbers can help you and your healthcare provider make informed decisions.

4. **Healthy Diet:** Adopt a heart-healthy diet rich in fruits, vegetables, whole grains, lean proteins, and healthy fats. Limit salt, cholesterol, trans fats, and saturated fats. Read food labels to assist you in making informed choices.

5. **Regular Exercise:** Make physical activity a regular part of your schedule. Aim for a combination of aerobic and strength-training exercises. Find activities you enjoy to stay motivated.

6. **Weight Management:** Maintain a healthy weight through balanced eating and regular physical activity. Heart health depends on achieving and maintaining a healthy weight.

7. **Stress Management:** Learn stress-reduction techniques such as deep breathing, meditation, mindfulness, or yoga to manage stress effectively. Reducing stress can benefit your heart health.

8. **Smoking Cessation:** If you smoke, quitting is one of the most significant steps you can take to improve heart health. To stop smoking, look for resources and help.

9. **Limit Alcohol:** If you consume alcohol, do so in moderation. Excessive alcohol intake can have negative effects on heart health.

10. **Quality Sleep:** Aim for 7-9 hours of quality sleep per night. Poor sleep can negatively impact your heart health.

11. **Medication Adherence:** If you're prescribed medications, take them as directed by your healthcare provider. Adhering to medication regimens is crucial for managing heart conditions.

12. **Screenings and Tests:** Follow your healthcare provider's recommendations for screenings and diagnostic tests based on your risk factors and medical history.

13. **Support System:** Maintain strong social connections and communicate with friends and family about your heart health journey. A support system can be invaluable.

14. **Emergency Preparedness:** Know the signs and symptoms of heart attacks and strokes. Have a plan for responding to cardiovascular emergencies.

15. **Advocacy:** Be an advocate for your own health. Ask questions, seek second opinions when needed, and actively participate in decisions about your heart health.

16. **Keep Learning:** Stay informed about heart health and emerging research. You can make more informed decisions regarding your health if you are well-informed.

17. **Consult Experts:** Work with healthcare providers, registered dietitians, and other experts to create a personalized plan for your heart health.

Empowering yourself for heart-healthy living is a commitment to a healthier, longer life with a strong and resilient heart. By making informed choices and taking proactive steps, you can protect your cardiovascular well-being and reduce the risk of heart disease.

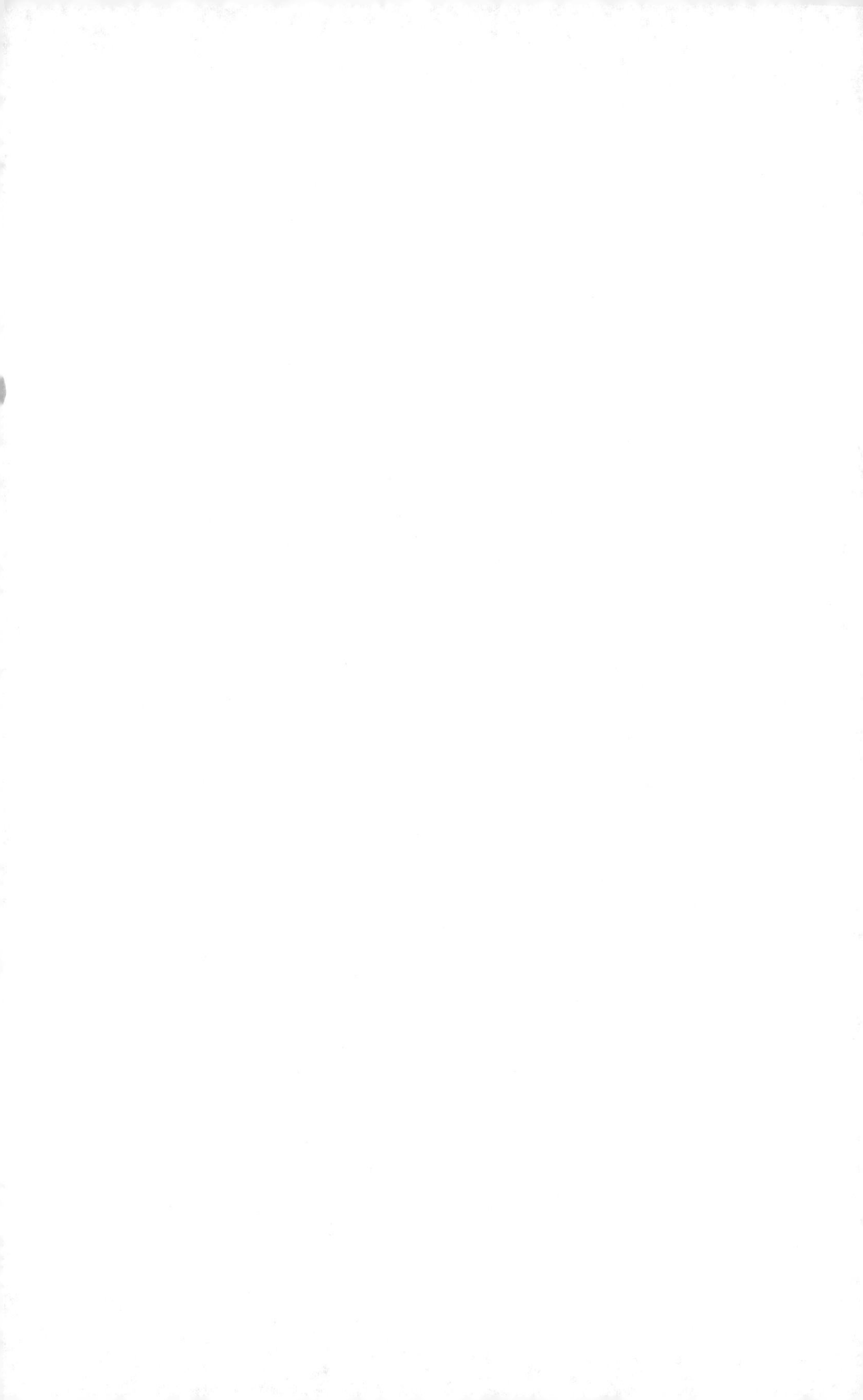

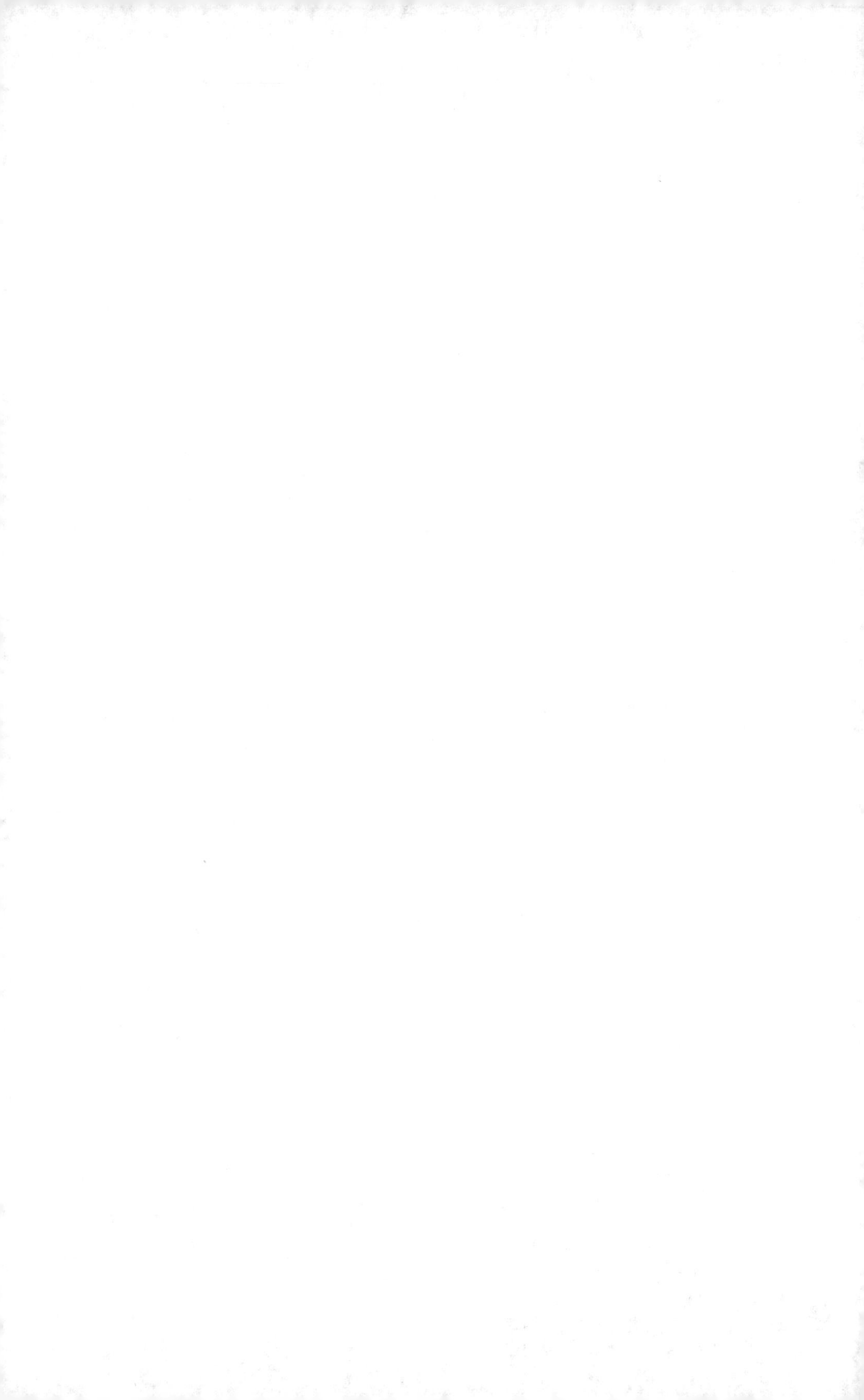